Healing the Heart, Soul, and Body

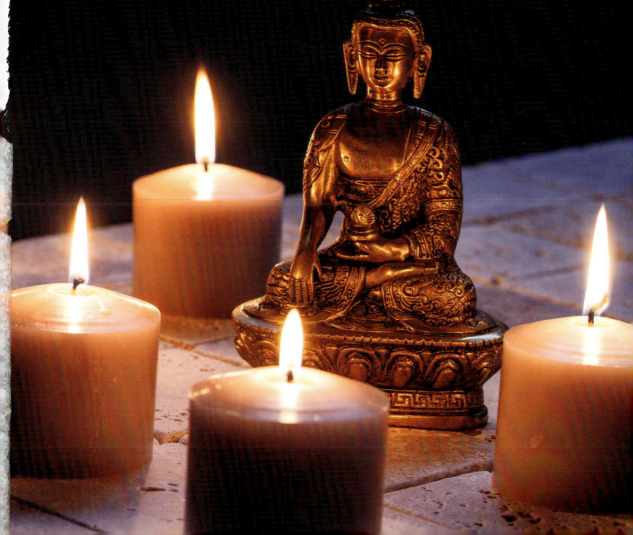

Healing the Heart, Soul, and Body

Spiritual Guidance and Transformative Inspiration from Yoga Leaders

Stephanie Spence
Foreword by Rolf Gates

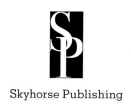

Skyhorse Publishing

Copyright © 2018, 2025 by Stephanie Spence
Foreword © 2018, 2025 by Rolf Gates

Previously published as *Yoga Wisdom*.

All rights reserved. No part of this book may be reproduced in any manner without the express written consent of the publisher, except in the case of brief excerpts in critical reviews or articles. All inquiries should be addressed to Skyhorse Publishing, 307 West 36th Street, 11th Floor, New York, NY 10018.

Skyhorse Publishing books may be purchased in bulk at special discounts for sales promotion, corporate gifts, fund-raising, or educational purposes. Special editions can also be created to specifications. For details, contact the Special Sales Department, Skyhorse Publishing, 307 West 36th Street, 11th Floor, New York, NY 10018 or info@skyhorsepublishing.com.

Skyhorse® and Skyhorse Publishing® are registered trademarks of Skyhorse Publishing, Inc.®, a Delaware corporation.

Visit our website at www.skyhorsepublishing.com.

10 9 8 7 6 5 4 3 2 1

Library of Congress Cataloging-in-Publication Data available on file.

Cover design by David Ter-Avanesyan
Cover illustration by Getty Images

Print ISBN: 978-1-5107-8380-5
Ebook ISBN: 978-1-5107-8387-4

Printed in China

Dedication

To Michael, with love and gratitude.
And to both of my daughters, with love.

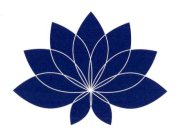

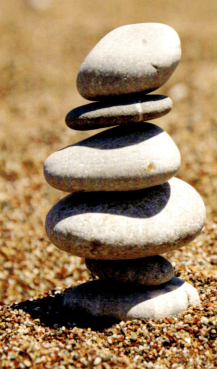

Contents

Author's Note to the Revised Edition ix

Foreword by Rolf Gates xi

Introduction 1

Chapter 1: Embracing Your Wake-up Call 5

Chapter 2: Getting on the Road 20

Chapter 3: Reading Your Life Road Map 35

Chapter 4: Staying Real 55

Chapter 5: Embracing the Potholes and Detours of Life 71

Chapter 6: Learning, Changing, and Growing 89

Chapter 7: Making Yoga Your Healthy
Life-Changing Tool 106

Chapter 8: Remaining Accountable 122

Chapter 9: How Yoga Helps You Trust Your
Own Inner Compass 141

Chapter 10: The Quest for Authenticity, Balance,
and Health 159

Chapter 11: You Arrive at Freedom 179

Acknowledgments 205

Contributors 207

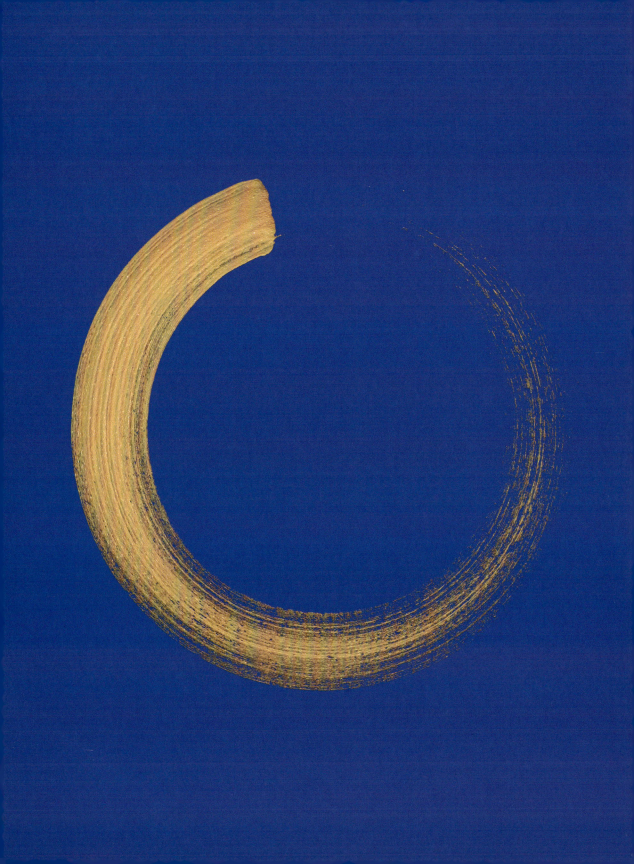

Author's Note to the Revised Edition

Since embarking on my transformative Yoga Road Trip and first sharing my insights in *Yoga Wisdom*, a previous edition of the book you are holding, the world is in pervasive and accelerated change. Recent societal upheavals and collective traumas have brought us to a pivotal juncture in our shared journey. Amid these shifting tides, one truth emerges clearly: the question is no longer whether healing is needed but how we, as individuals and as a collective, choose to embrace it.

At the heart of this healing lies a nurturing force within us all—the essence of our collective consciousness. This force embodies the sacred feminine: a deep well of compassion, intuition, and resilience. True healing transcends the personal; it is a collective necessity. The traumas of our time—political, social, and personal—are urgent cries for balance, urging us to realign our inner and outer worlds.

As a yoga scholar, I see yoga as more than a practice; it is an ancient pathway to reconnect with the wisdom of the body and the resilience of the spirit. Yoga invites us to go beyond the surface, to explore the depths of who we are—beyond trauma, beyond fragmentation, and into wholeness. It offers a sanctuary where we can cultivate mindfulness, honor the body's memories, and learn to breathe into our discomfort with the gentle curiosity of an inner mother.

Through yoga, we begin to dissolve the hardened identities we've built for survival—those that isolate and defend us. Instead, we open ourselves to vulnerability and reflection, allowing the sacred feminine within to awaken. This sacred force guides us in collective healing. In the stillness of asana and the silence between breaths, we find courage to acknowledge our wounds, honor our grief, and transform pain into growth.

My own healing journey remains rooted in yoga, a practice I've now experienced in over sixty countries. Each place and its inhabitants have deepened my understanding of how universally humankind is embracing yoga's teachings. This shared embrace is a testament to how far we've come and the promise of what lies ahead.

I am continually inspired by our shared capacity for resilience, reflection, and renewal. May we all find the courage to embrace this capacity and move forward together with hope and strength.

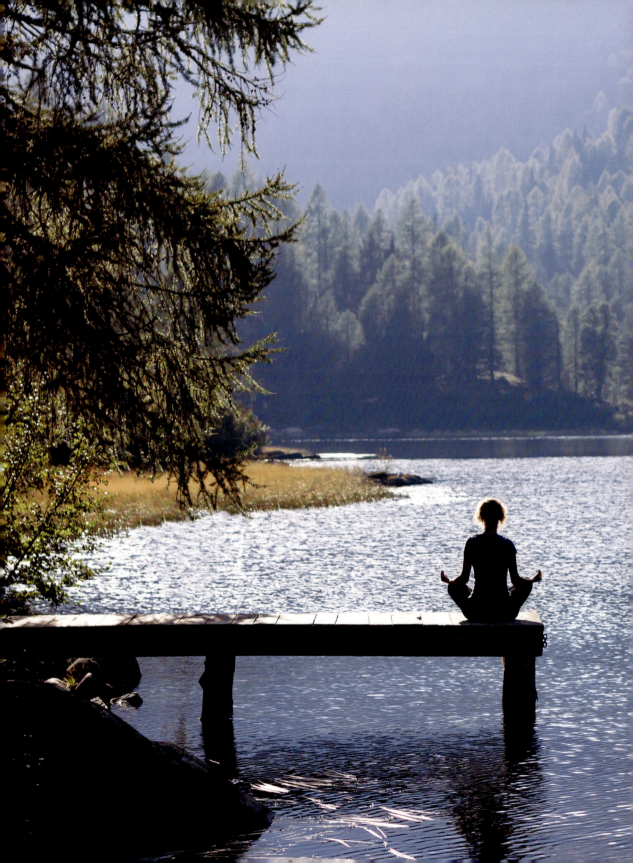

Foreword by Rolf Gates

I read once that a single-cell organism can either grow or it can defend itself; it cannot do both at the same time. Stephanie Spence has written beautifully about what this means through a human life. For a time, she was defined by the need to defend herself. Then one day things changed. She found safety. She found connection. She felt the Sacred. She found sanctuary. Held by kindness and compassion, she was able to put her burden down. Those who held her taught her how to hold herself, and she in turn has learned to hold others. Today, her life is defined by the possibility of growth. Hers is now the hero's journey.

I met Stephanie on that journey some years ago as she was beginning the series of interviews that would become this book. She came to Santa Cruz and interviewed me with the intelligence and joy I have come to associate with yoga practice. There is something that happens when you combine getting a second chance at life with the practices of awakening that is unmistakable. People just radiate. She was not yet sure what she wanted to do with her interviews, but she was clear about her intention, which was to support others as they chose the path of Yoga. She still embodies this clarity today.

Believing that sanctuary is something we choose in the silent private space of our hearts and create in the loud colorful space of our togetherness, Stephanie has written a book about what we choose for ourselves and what we create together. Believing that learning is one part listening and one part teaching, Stephanie has written a book that combines her voice with many others. Knowing that this book will be a joy to those who pick it up, it is my honor to welcome you to its sunlit shores.

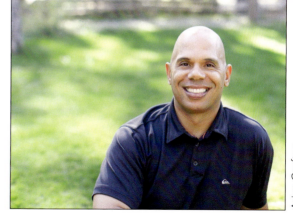

Arica Grafton

Namaste, Rolf

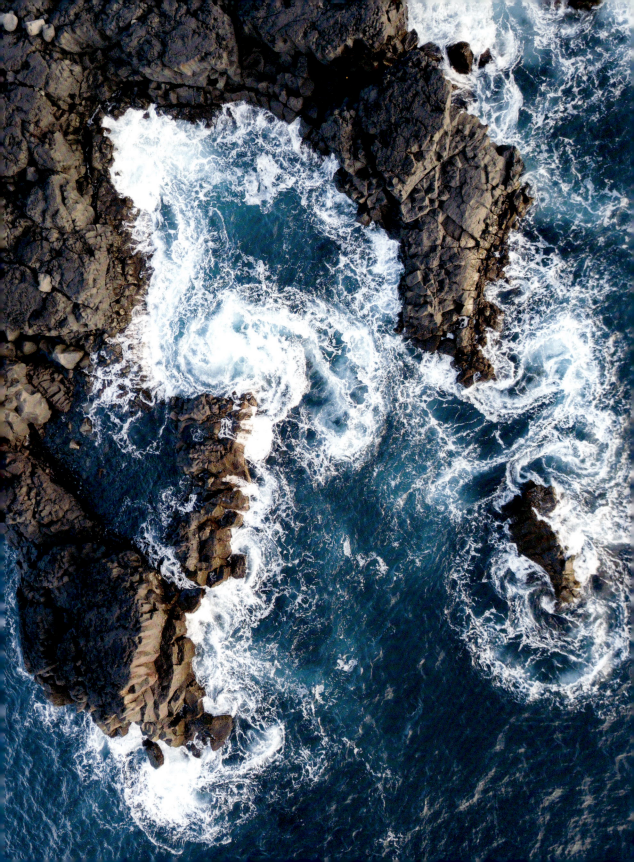

Introduction

The setting: a luxurious villa on the Caribbean island of St. Barts. A wife and husband, along with several of his clients, are partying on a terrace overlooking the glittering ocean and sun-kissed beach. They flew in from Pittsburgh aboard his private jet that morning. The woman seems to have it all—she's a self-made success story, wife, and mother. But beneath her mask of contentment and complicity, she hides a terrible secret: the price she's paying for this glamorous life is that she is living a lie. Their friends and acquaintances would say that she and her rich, powerful husband of twenty-five years never argue. Well, *she* doesn't argue. Why? She is terrified of being bullied, verbally dismissed, and belittled.

As usual, she is expected to entertain her husband's guests, which means fulfilling their every desire—no matter how illegal. Submissive and compliant, her everyday mantra. Soon, the revelers want to kick things up a notch with Thai Stick, some of the best opium-laced marijuana money can buy. And they expect her to join in.

She takes the Stick, feels her stomach rebel. Her mind screams in protest. She brings the smoldering joint to her lips . . . and hesitates. Her husband, waiting his turn, nods for her to take a hit.

She parts her lips, ready to obey. *Wait. What am I doing?* she thinks. *Selling her soul. Giving herself away.*

Putting toxic substances into her body because her husband expects her to be the life of the party. *She drops the Stick in a most deliberate way, oblivious to the gasps and protests. No. No more.*

She is done with drugs, drinking, and ass-kissing. Ignoring one man's dash to grab the Stick, now rolling across the patio, she turns to the man who had once vowed to honor and love her. His mouth moves, trying to form words in his shocked outrage.

Before his drug-hazed mind can produce the vitriol he so clearly wants to spew, she blurts out, "I want a divorce."

A startled hush falls over everyone as they wait for his reaction. She's prepared for the worst of his explosive temper. Instead of denigrating her, threatening her, or pretending that he cares, he simply walks out of the villa. Minutes later, she hears him drive away.

She excuses herself and holes up in one of the guest rooms to await his return. The waiting is its own torture, and it's for nothing. She finds out that he boarded his jet and left her behind.

But he wasn't done. The following day, he sends her an email with only one sentence: "Your life as you know it will never be the same."

My name is Stephanie Spence, a.k.a. Yoga Road Trip Girl, and that wife was me. That brave, bold declaration was only the beginning. As any survivor of abuse, whether physical, emotional, or mental, knows, you can't go from living as a shell of your former self to empowered in a day, a week, a month. For me, it's an ongoing journey of triumphs and failures, of heartbreak and joy.

I set off on my new life with nothing but a rental car and the clothes on my back and slowly rebuilt my life with the only lifeline I knew: yoga.

My daily yoga practice grew into so much more than perfecting a pose. Yoga became transformative, teaching me to live a fearless, authentic life of purpose and potential.

When I felt alone, it reminded me that I was part of a world-wide community. When I was hard on myself for falling out of a pose, it reminded me that this is a practice, not an end goal. When I felt powerless to master a pose, it reminded me to surrender to what is. When I hurt, it helped me to heal. And when I did master a pose at last, it applauded my strength—and showed me that I am a warrior at heart who can save *myself*.

When we are ready to grow, the Universe puts "coincidences" on our path to help us or send us in the right direction. These can be people, places, or events that your soul attracts into your life to help you evolve to higher consciousness or place emphasis on something going on in your life. Synchronistically, I met spiritual teacher Gahl Sasson through my yoga studio. My session with Gahl was infused with Kabbalah, the ancient Jewish mystical interpretation of the Bible. Gahl's depth of wisdom and devotion inspired me to deepen my spiritual practice, along with my yoga practice. I devoured the exercises in his book, *A Wish Can Change Your Life*. Starting from the first chapter, I had visual, emotional, and physical confirmation that the book was working. This was unlike any other self-help book I had read. I immediately saw results. For the first time in my life, I had a clear direction for my future.

By the time I finished the book, I knew that my dharma, my soul purpose, was to educate and inspire as many people as I could to try yoga and embrace it as a way of life. I loaded up a rented RV and headed on a month-long journey I dubbed the "Yoga Road Trip." Waking up daily in my moving cocoon of yoga, I felt powerful and free. My morning ritual of writing and playing house in my adopted home electrified my soul. It dawned on me that this was the first house I had ever picked out and lived in that was truly my own.

Whether my morning meditation was in a shabby trailer park, busy parking lot, or overlooking the ocean, I had a space that was all mine. I embodied the new freedom and adventure I had always longed for but had never been able to manifest on my own.

As I made my 4,000-mile pilgrimage from Southern California all the way up the West Coast and into Canada, I had a simple mission: video-interview and practice with a different yoga teacher every day. Instead of solely words and pictures on my blog, I hoped the moving images would resonate on a more intimate level with the viewers, bringing them closer to these wise souls, my experience, and me. Hungry for emotional connection, I believed the world of online sharing would resonate with the yearning for kinship that I believe is at the root of all social media. I pictured the blog more as a vlog (video log) from a vision I had while in Savasana. I also wanted to capture their wisdom and enlightenment to help me discover a part of myself I had never known. The me that I was before life taught me destructive love. I had never learned to listen to and trust my spiritual self, the wise and loving voice of my intuition.

SPIRITUAL WARRIOR WISDOM

I reclaimed my lost self on the road. I understood for the first time how to thrive instead of merely survive. I regained my unique power and my voice. And most important, I had a road map for physical, mental, and spiritual health to give others. The impressive souls I met on my Yoga Road Trip, and those I have engaged with as I continue my journey, are at the heart of this book.

I became a Spiritual Warrior when I embraced the understanding that I had to crash so I could transform my life. I scoured the globe to find top yoga teachers, truly authentic givers, who make yoga a way of life just as I do. They have huge hearts and simple wisdom driven by compassion, experience, and kindness. We all hope *Healing the Heart, Soul, and Body* inspires the whole world to embrace yoga as a way of life, one person at a time.

Healing the Heart, Soul, and Body takes you on the road of life with people who are full of self-love and radiating balance, so you can create that for yourself. Once you meet these life instructors, you can manifest everything you need to make a difference in your life and the lives of those around you.

Physically showing up on your yoga mat is just the beginning. With determination and patience, the real secrets and power of yoga come with time. We're here to inspire you to not only show up for class, but to become a yogi, too—a yoga devotee full of love and light.

It's time to unleash the *Spiritual Warrior* inside you.

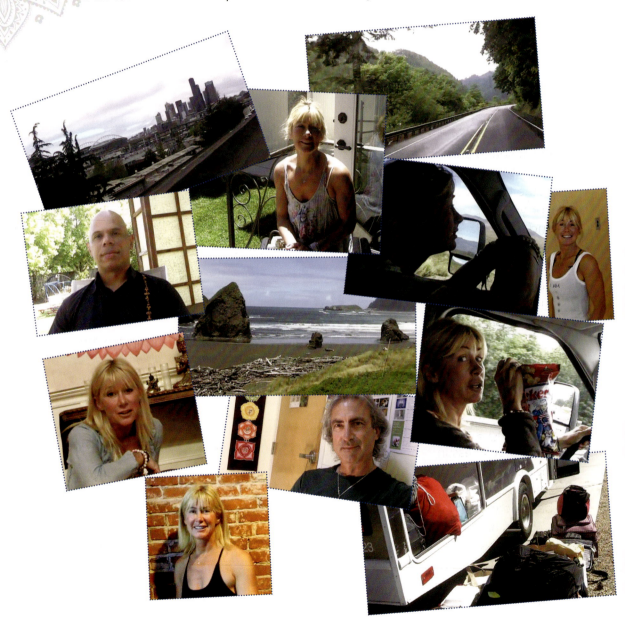

CHAPTER 1

Embracing Your Wake-up Call

I read somewhere that every marriage reaches a point when it feels as though it's going to unravel. I'm not sure if that's true or not. All I know is that I thought my husband and I were different. We were friends. Best friends.

We'd met twenty-five years earlier as neighbors in Houston, Texas. I believed at the time that our bond would get us through any challenges life heaved at us. For years, it did, with failed ventures and poverty, moving across the country, and many dark years of infertility. I finally achieved my fondest goal: having a beautiful baby girl. Then, after all the struggles with the first one, while not even trying, good fortune smiled upon me, and I became pregnant a second time. I had an optimistic attitude, even when we were so poor that a block of government-assisted Reagan Cheese sat in the fridge, and I was rolling pennies to buy toilet paper.

Like many entrepreneurs, my husband tried numerous ways to make money. I supported him emotionally and, at times, financially. I believed in "for better or worse." Sometimes, we could pay our bills just fine, then we'd hit a wall and couldn't. This roller coaster went on for years.

Clearly, we were going nowhere in Houston. He had exhausted all avenues of producing a steady income, including cleaning carpets at night while trying to build a business in the oil industry during the day. My husband's falling out with his business partner finally put the nail in the coffin, and we had to crawl back to his hometown, Pittsburgh, with our tails between our legs and live in his parents' basement while we looked for work.

Upon arrival, my husband jumped on an opportunity a distant relative offered him. He became an overnight success, and, just like that, the money started flooding in. I created a wellness magazine, *Health & Fitness*. It too was immediately successful. Years later, I created a second magazine, *Pittsburgh NOW*, designated as the city's official visitors guide. We were "Seen Column" darlings in the local newspapers and glossy society magazines. After years of struggling, we had reinvented ourselves as quite the power couple.

I had what appeared to be a fairy-tale life with the perfect family and career. I had a whole slew of smiling family photos, mementos from world travels, and many awards from my career. All of this sat on a bookcase crammed with self-help books. Holy crap, a bookcase full of self-help books? Yeah, I was searching. I would desperately pore through each new book, believing it to be the one that would explain what was calling to me from my consciousness—the element of my life that was missing and creating a bigger and bigger hole in my soul. Despite my self-made success, I was not the decision maker of my life.

I had succumbed to accepting the hand I had been dealt. This included living in a town I had a love-hate relationship with. I pasted on an interested, happy face, pretending fascination with my husband's clients and colleagues—whose only intellectual contribution included sports and the awful weather. I was on autopilot, simply doing what my husband told me to do for the sake of the almighty dollar. I was in deep despair, and there wasn't even enough light in my darkness to see that I had simply checked out of my own life.

Sure, I had all the outward trappings of success, but I was a fraud—and terrified that I would be found out. Most painfully, at the same time, I was aware of my amazing soul whenever I was with my two daughters, working on my magazines with my team and clients, and not around my husband. I knew my soul was filled with love and wisdom, and that I was capable of more in all aspects of my life.

But knowing that didn't help. Even worse, my marriage had disintegrated into two people living in the same house but barely speaking to each other. How could this be? We had managed to weather the many years of our financial instabilities and five years of infertility. I loved being a mother and all that it entailed, but not being a single parent. By now, though, our rare conversations were superficial, or focused on only two things: him or work.

We may have been physically in the same room, but we were emotionally alone. We were busy, too busy to evaluate our increasingly disconnected relationship. If we weren't busy, we just didn't know how to even begin a discussion.

I know now that I ignored many of the classic red flags and dismissed the growing dissonance between us. He had moved out of our bedroom to the spare bedroom down the hall, giving me no reason. Taking the rejection personally, I fell into an even deeper well, drowning in insecurity and hopeless abandonment.

However, it takes two to tango, and I accept accountability for my part in the demise of our relationship. I used exercise for time to myself to be away from my husband's chaos. When it came to focusing my energy, his needs, raising my

6　❁　HEALING THE HEART, SOUL, AND BODY

daughters, and helping others through my magazines took all of my time. Healthy people are mindful of self-care. I didn't think about myself and my needs.

When I mustered up the courage to ask if he would hold my hand, his response chilled me to bone: he laughed. He obviously didn't understand that holding hands and touch were relationship basics. His rejection of my simple request for an emotional connection demoralized me beyond repair. My heart was no longer in the marriage.

In the most spineless attempt to declare my unhappiness, I turned the focus of my own concern to concern for him. I explained that he seemed ill from the stress of the business. I also suggested that we see a family therapist. He said that would be impossible, for fear someone would find out. Instead, we agreed to go away alone to St. Barts. Much to my surprise and disappointment, he brought along clients.

St. Barts sealed the deal. I was done. After that first ominous email, his second one seemed more sinister: he declared that I needed an "intervention." I knew I needed to overcome my dependency on the prescription sleep aid Ambien, so getting professional help seemed a reasonable first step for getting my divorce. I believe now that his intent was to reset me so he could get his old girl back.

When I arrived home from St. Barts, my intervention began. Ushered to a therapist's office, she informed me that we were going to embark on a new beginning.

The word *beginning* has such a hopeful and inspirational feel, right? Yet, on the day I acquiesced to my intervention, the concept of beginning felt strangely menacing. I had allowed myself to be signed up for a therapist chosen by my controlling and domineering husband.

Since a small child, I'd been trained to obey abusers rather than think for myself. To, in fact, accept dysfunction as normal. In my husband's case, I'd been drinking his Kool-Aid for years. Sure, in the beginning, our marriage seemed good, but then I began to see behavioral signs that scared me. In the space of a few hours, his moods would swing wildly from excited to unable to get off the couch. Being angry or hiding in his bathroom became the norm. He always suffered numerous physical complaints that needed attention. Our friendship bond turned into me navigating the ups and downs of an undiagnosed bipolar person.

I used to tell myself during our many years together that he was "passionate," certainly not bipolar or bullying or narcissistic, and that his actions were inspired by love and concern for me. When he said, "You're sick and need help," in an

EMBRACING YOUR WAKE-UP CALL

angry, threatening voice, I fell silent. Too afraid to cross him, I did what I was told. Partly because I did need help—but not of the kind he imagined.

It never entered my mind to first hire an attorney, seek counsel from the clergy, confide in a close friend or my parents, to help me think this divorce thing through. The idea of telling anyone felt embarrassing, even humiliating. I look back now and realize that I did have a couple of friends who would have been good sounding boards. But I never bothered anyone with my problems, ever. Nor did I share the intimate details of my marriage with anyone. The truth is, I never thought past summoning the courage to say I wanted a divorce.

Like most days in Pittsburgh, it was cold and gray when we arrived at my new therapist's office for our first session. I had no clue what therapy entailed. I just knew I had to be there or suffer the consequences.

In my naïveté, I assumed that my therapist had my well-being in mind. After all, she's a professional, an unbiased person who would listen to my side of the story. I had no reason to choose my words carefully; it never occurred to me to protect myself.

I should have grown concerned when she started speaking to me as she would to a child. We discussed my use of Ambien. I told her I couldn't sleep without it. With Ambien (and thus, sleep), I had no drama, no stress, no angry husband, no fear, no nothing. Upon waking, my feet would once again hit the floor, and I'd go until I dropped at the end of a busy day. Productive? You bet. That's what my life was about. Working. Achieving. Perfecting.

She asked where and how I could obtain a constant supply. "It's easy," I said. "When I run out, I track down the doctor on my husband's payroll." Never once did this doctor seem concerned about how much I took. On several occasions, I confessed my fear that I was addicted. He'd smile, pat me on the shoulder, and say, "You're only dependent." I trusted him.

I believed myself the epitome of health. After all, front and center as the CEO and editor of the popular *Health & Fitness* magazine, I spent my time helping others lead a healthy life. An avid runner, I balanced that with yoga and ate clean. I only drank alcohol socially. I didn't shop too much, eat donuts, or do anything to excess. My worst flaw was a propensity for cussing.

My husband started screaming that this wasn't about him when I revealed that he took it also. After the therapist escorted him out of the room, she told me that she had experience with this type of situation. She let out a long breath that sounded more like a sigh of boredom, leaned in close, and whispered, "It's not easy being married to a successful man."

What? That's the big revelation? My Ambien dependency is driven by my emotional resistance to having a successful husband? I knew I was in trouble.

She explained my options. I could come every week for seven or so years to address my emotional resistance issues and my Ambien dependency. With no reference point or voice, I didn't push back. As I sat in silence, she went on to say that I could go away for a month to a center she'd already selected. Did I have emotional resistance issues? Maybe. All I know is, I simply couldn't articulate what I wanted and needed in my life. I was stuck.

Convinced I was to blame for everything wrong in my world, I jumped at the chance to solve my issues in a month. Who wouldn't? I'd had my wake-up call. I was going to get help.

Within days, my therapist and I were on my husband's private jet en route to a treatment center in the Arizona desert. Little did I know that an escort was unusual. I was clueless, but ready.

SPIRITUAL WARRIOR WISDOM

At that time, my only healthy coping tool was yoga. I had been doing yoga for a long time, but I desperately needed to take it deeper. It was essential to find ways to utilize yoga as more than a fitness tool. A trusted yoga friend would have been invaluable. If I could have chosen an authentic and wise teacher to call on and ask for advice, I would have called Seane Corn.

Seane teaches all over the world and is one of the most recognized names in yoga, but as you will see when you meet her, she is very down-to-earth. The real deal. Seane shared recently that although she too had been practicing and teaching yoga a very long time, her father's death gave her the wake-up call to take her practice deeper. Seane shares, "Yoga has taught me that life happens. It's amazing and it's incredible and it kicks your ass backwards."

Seane Corn

"Yoga is a creative expression. Creativity grows and changes. I'm only one aspect and color of a massive tapestry, and sometimes I can only see what is in front of me (and miss the bigger picture). I'm amazed at what's happening in the world of yoga. But I also get concerned. Is it going to get diluted, become a parody of itself? And then I think, well, it's been around for thousands of years, and I'm only on a small part of its pathway.

What that means, then, is that I'm accountable to be authentic and in integrity so that what I'm contributing is mindful and positive.

Yoga has taught me that life happens. It's amazing and it's incredible and it kicks your ass backwards. It's completely unpredictable, and no one is guaranteed an effortless pathway. It's taught me that there are tools we can utilize, so that when life does happen, and we experience loss, oppression, or unimaginable heartache, we can stay present to the experience. We can navigate it and make choices that are grounded, compassionate, fair, and love-filled.

That is what yoga has taught me . . . *you cannot bypass the challenges of life*, but you can learn to change your perspective so that every experience—the light and the shadow—provides opportunities for spiritual maturity, wisdom, and growth."

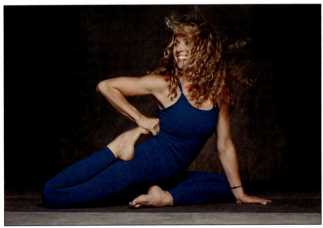

Norman Seeff

Opportunity. What an optimistic word. I was certainly lacking in spiritual maturity and am grateful that the program I was in at the treatment facility focused on just that. I was determined to become whole. Part of that was learning about vulnerability. My friend, Chris Loebsack, also wore the mask of a person who had it all together. Think for a moment if you are wearing a mask now.

Chris Loebsack

"There is strength in vulnerability!

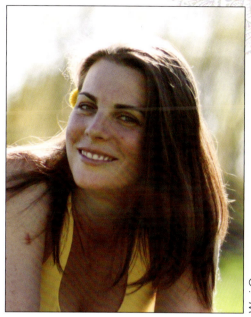

For a long time, I had grown to believe that to be whole you needed to be strong in all ways. I took this to heart in ways that didn't always serve. I built walls around me so high that I couldn't see the horizon. I was the person everyone turned to, but no one seemed to ask about. Rightfully so. Why would anyone check in on someone who has it together all the time? I still found myself disconnected.

Today, I am more at home in my heart and stronger for it. I can listen more and react less. Yoga has taught me to embrace the nature of who I am in all my expressions and to love each aspect of my being. Self-love is essential. This is different from self-esteem. Not everything I have done is worthy of esteem, yet at the end of the day, I can reflect and grow, and love the life I have and who I am within it.

Life and the yoga practice are like music. You start with learning the basic notes, you progress to scales and chords, and the more you practice the fundamentals, the more confidence you get. When you learn the framework, you have the freedom to play the music of your heart. The same is true in the body and mind. We learn poses and build upon the fundamentals of the breath, focus, alignment, muscular energy, and subtle awareness. As we come to the practice again and again, the music of the body and heart has the opportunity to unfold. We get out what we are willing to put into it. It is an incredible step-by-step journey that can send you forward into boundless possibilities.

Yoga has helped me overcome many physical, mental, and emotional challenges. The tools present in the practice are like the brushes available to a painter. You can choose the one that helps you make the desired stroke for the right effect at that time. There are times we have to wipe the canvas clean and start over to create the picture we desire for our lives."

How scary that seemed to me at the time: to wipe the canvas clean. What would that look like? Fear of the unknown is what holds us back from even the smallest steps. Like Chris, I always prided myself on never needing anyone's help. Now was different. I was going to have to learn how to be vulnerable. Was that possible?

What would it have been like to have heard my friend, Dhanpal-Donna Quesada, say that "we're on this spiritual journey even if we don't know it" and be able to stop, breathe, and just restart. I had been studying Buddhism, but I wasn't practicing it. It became much more important to devote time to my spiritual life. Do you cultivate that in your life?

Dhanpal-Donna Quesada

"We heal ourselves first and then awaken to the call to help others in the way only we can . . . because we've been through it. *Our trials and heartaches are the seedlings that unfold our spiritual journey.* They nudge us into a search for the deeper meaning of it all until we find ourselves on a path of healing, which is one and the same as the path to what the yogis call union.

Yoga is a vehicle to bring us to a sense of connection and wholeness within ourselves, and communion with the divine. It's about that calling deep within the heart to go higher, to go within, to go beyond the trials, and even the thrills, of the mundane.

The most important part of a human being's life is the journey back to the soul— and we're on this spiritual journey even if we don't yet know it. It is often the heaviest blows that awaken us to the urgency to find some sweetness.

We've all had our own dark night of the soul. The struggle pushes us, as if from the depths of the deepest and darkest waters, to try to find our way back to the light. Our desperation to try to find an answer to it all is a necessary part of it. It's a wonderful wake-up call. Don't feel that you are being punished by life. While everybody else might seem happy-go-lucky, they are probably still sleeping, while you are being nudged awake. The suffering is an inevitable part of the polarity that brings us back.

In my own longing to find my way through the murkiness, I came across the same messages again and again, no matter the tradition, that the light is within. And when this light is shining, the darkness on the *outside* suddenly appears differently, which is to say, the worries that used to bring us down lose their power over us. That light doesn't stay on by itself, which is why things like meditation and yoga are called practices. The challenges never stop, and so the need to practice never ends. Once we begin to slack off, the light begins to dim.

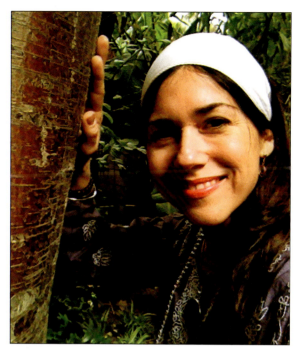

This journey back to spirit is never about being perfect or having our lives go as planned. Embrace yourself in your totality—start where you are, anew at every moment. The path to self-acceptance is one and the same as the path to the divine. This journey, this life, your human experience, is about being authentically who you are."

I'm continually astonished at the expansiveness of yoga and how it can deal with emotional *and* physical elements. I promise you that learning a new thing or two about diving into authenticity could dramatically change your life. At the time of my wake-up call, I was hiding behind perfecting.

Talking with someone like Kathryn Budig, who knows that *life isn't about perfecting*, would have helped me at that time. I could have drawn inspiration from her courage. The kind of inspiration I'm talking about is, for example, when she says yoga is *". . . a safe place of honesty where I can look my demons in the face."*

There's an incredible moment when you realize that growth might be easier than you think. Consider scheduling time in your day, knowing that it might mean getting rid of something else—like sitting in front of a TV—to roll out your mat. Your practice will change, as Kathryn Budig shares, when your perspective does.

EMBRACING YOUR WAKE-UP CALL

Kathryn Budig

"Yoga taught me that I can't be defined by my physicality and that life isn't about perfecting—it's a constant practice. I used to think I was as good as my asana. I thought my physical execution of the postures externally defined my level of dedication to the practice. I now know that yoga isn't about perfecting poses, but about finding a beautiful balance in our lives. I strive to learn and be stronger every day but am better in tune with the more subtle needs through meditation and my personal offerings.

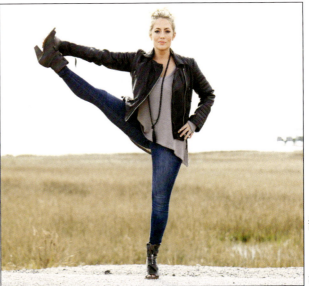

Cheyenne Ellis

My motto in life is 'Aim true.' It came from my love of Artemis, the goddess of the hunt. She inspired me to sport a gold arrow around my neck because it reminded me of her strength, and that I can always hit my mark when I set intention, follow what makes my heart beat, and aim true. The arrow is a reminder that I can cut through any obstacles, that I have power, beauty, and the ability to choose love over fear every moment of my life.

My yoga mat is an island of solace where I can go to strip away the layers of my ego and fear-based decisions and see what's actually going on. It's a safe place of honesty where I can look my demons in the face and put my big girl panties on."

A safe place is something we all need. Create that for yourself. Although, no matter how safe things could be in any given moment, unexpected challenges will arise. Things happen to us in addition to our choices. Life isn't always about our behaviors. Sometimes an illness is the entry point to starting a yoga practice.

Julie Smerdon

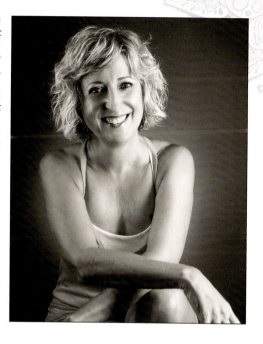

"Love your body. I was diagnosed with an autoimmune disorder at the age of thirteen, and my response to that was to try and have complete control over my body and my health by using a grueling fitness regimen. Even my early years of yoga were spent in a style of practice that was quite harsh. Eventually, I learned that my body, even with its substantial limitations (I've had heart surgery, my colon removed, and I've nearly died twice!), is a masterpiece. When I was able to love and accept and be grateful for all that my body had seen me through, it changed everything for me. I can have the strong physical practice I've always loved, but it can be joyful and life-enhancing rather than punitive and harsh.

Inquire rather than judge. It's so easy to make a decision about someone based on what we *think* we see, and I've been wrong more times than I care to admit. Judging keeps me from genuinely knowing and tuning in, not only to my students, but to anyone I'm in a relationship with. Relationship is the highest spiritual practice there is. Asking questions and really listening to the answers help me to be present, which means that I can honestly see and recognize the people around me.

I've had a lot of challenge in my life. Some of it I chose for myself, and some of it has been the hand I was dealt. Hard times happen, there is no doubt about that. The ebb and flow of life contains moments of great joy and expansion, and moments of deep sadness and contraction. But through yoga I've come to have a strong belief that life is good, and that even in the darkest times, there is a *loving* intelligence and order to things."

Julie's grace and wisdom inspire me to this day. One of the best ways you can lean in to your greatness is to surround yourself with people like Julie and Hope Zvara, who will encourage you to make changes only you can make.

Hope Zvara

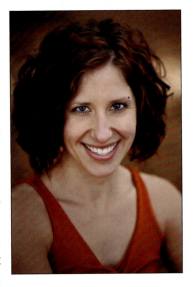

"Yoga has taught me a lot about what I am made of, a lot about my true inner voice and how to speak it with compassion and honesty. Yoga has taught me a lot about how not to be afraid of what I have inside of me, and also to share it with those around me.

Yoga is more about what we experience off the mat than what we will ever experience on it.

Everything we experience on our mat is a mirror image for how we live in our everyday lives: how we are moving, how we are breathing, how we are acting and reacting to the things, people, and situations around us. To me, this is why we need yoga, the kind of yoga I know, the yoga that forces us to look in the mirror, see who we are, and then asks us to make a change only we can make. That change, that is the yoga that I know. That mirror has restructured my thinking from self-destructive, self-denial, and self-hate to self-love, self-respect, and self-discovery.

Yoga also teaches you to act in a yogic way, a nonharming, mindful, purposeful way. My yoga mat, however, has become my place to step back and take a breath. It has been a place for my body to become toned and flexible and strong, but what is a physical body without a healthy soul and mind?

Before yoga, I had been in battle with myself through depression, addiction of various kinds consisting of a cocktail of eating disorders, drugs, alcohol, self-loathing, and thoughts of suicide because I didn't think I was worthy. Yoga brought back my self-worth, my zest for life. Yoga reminded me that there was and still is purpose for me. Yoga forced me in a very powerful and present way to face my fears, my anxieties. Yoga made me face . . . myself."

Have you ever noticed that, when something is on your mind, you see synchronicities? I didn't know anyone when I lived in Pittsburgh who had the courage to share the trauma in their life. Many people experience trauma, as you'll see with Ananda Tinio, but most are reluctant to share, for a variety of reasons. Here, though, she shares a tendency I knew all too well: self-criticism.

Ananda Tinio

"Yoga healed me when I was most broken and vulnerable, and in the constant connection it gives me with others, it continues to heal me.

I experienced a series of traumas culminating in a nervous breakdown. I found myself at Laughing Lotus Yoga Center every day, weeping silently, wanting the fellowship, but running away at the first hint of conversation. Until slowly, I came into the fold.

Yoga's requisite self-investigation has enabled me to hone in on the crux of my internal struggle and root cause of personal suffering: I do not trust my inner voice.

A punitive critic presides over my mind that dominates my internal monologue and debilitates action, freedom, creativity, and happiness. I have no faith that answers exist inside of me, so I seek external validation, looking for external cures for the internal malady of spiritual impoverishment. Somewhere along the timeline of my life, I picked up messages from family, culture, etc., and internalized feelings of inadequacy. These internalized feelings developed into deep-seated, subconscious beliefs, giving birth to that cruel inner critic that serves to discount the truth and validity of my own experience and intuition.

My root feelings of unworthiness played out in the dramas of chronic substance abuse, self-mutilation, an eating disorder, anger, depression, divorce, and disastrous interpersonal relationships; the positive consequence of such behavior was a long, circuitous journey of recovery leading to yoga.

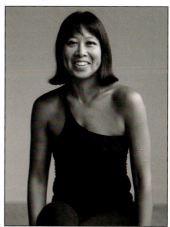

Over the years, yoga practice has taught me to detach from the relentless barrage of negative thoughts, helping me gain perspective and awareness with regard to over-identifying with self-criticism. I remind myself not to believe everything I think, but the critical voice fights hard to survive. Yoga has taught me that happiness (true, unadulterated happiness) is also a choice that requires constant work and cultivation (of authenticity rather than false positivity), discipline and vigilance, and personal accountability. I am ultimately responsible for my own rehabilitation, peace, and happiness."

When you find yourself repeating old patterns, get to your yoga mat. Get to a class that resonates with you. I would have loved to have met Ananda or Cindy Lusk when I was suffering, to be able to relate to someone. Smile in the understanding that you are not alone. We understand you.

Cindy Lusk

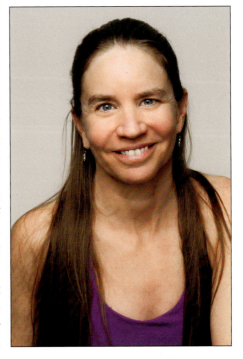

"Many seeds are planted in the garden of our life. Some seem to drift in from elsewhere, some we plant ourselves, and yoga philosophy tells us some are like seeds dormant from last year's garden. Some seeds grow as the conditions are right and we actively nurture them or unconsciously encourage them. Or they may be dormant for many years, until the circumstances are just right for them to sprout.

So it is with yoga. You have a choice about what you cultivate in the garden of your life. If you pause to consider and carefully choose, you can plant a seed that could change the whole trajectory of your life.

The conditions must be right for that seed to take hold. Yoga asana is an entryway. It is a way to engage our life force, our prana. It is also a context in which we can start to watch our minds. On the mat, we can observe how our habitual thought and behavior patterns emerge: how we work with pain and frustration. Do we listen? Are we competitive, or do we give up too easily?

As we start watching our minds and bodies, we begin to become more present. Some space emerges—the witness, the Seer, is there to facilitate the pause. We observe how the seeds begin to sprout, and we see that we have a great deal of freedom to pause and consciously decide: Which seeds do we want to cultivate? Can we take responsibility for the garden of our life?

Everything now present in our lives is there because we participated in cultivating it. Learn to pause and choose which seeds to plant and consciously tend in your garden.

Do you feel connected? Do you sense there is more to your life? Through practice, you can learn to exercise your freedom and cultivate the garden of your life that brings more connection, creates more beauty into the world, yields more love, and reflects your heart's truest desire."

Looking back, I now see that I had seeds ready to sprout, but because they were under my mounds of despair, I was unable to see how I had *participated in cultivating* the situation I was in. Fear kept me from cultivating my own happiness. I had given up on myself.

Living in fear sucks. If you need help, reach out, tell someone. You're not alone. There are varying degrees of fear. Even subtle degrees of detachment, lack of accountability, or "tools" like excessive busyness could be keeping you living a fear-based life. The hard part is taking that first step. Once you have, the Universe will conspire to help you. It's important to remember that there are people, resources, and organizations that can help. Once you've gotten clear about needing help, yoga could be one of many tools you use to heal and design a life in which you can thrive.

When you find yourself amidst your own wakeup call, yoga is a proven tool that helps. It's also important to understand your options for charting your path forward, or adjusting it if you've hit a roadblock. So, looking back, here is some warrior wisdom I gleaned from my experience:

1. Before blurting out something that could potentially impact the rest of your life, consult with someone: an attorney, clergy, or a local support group.

2. Call a friend or a family member, and ask for a confidential conversation. If you know someone in a similar situation, all the better. If you're afraid that no one will understand or believe you, sit down right now at your computer and search your situation in the form of a question. There are plenty of confidential resources out there for you.

3. If you want to change your life, first consider that you can.

4. If you're stressed, yoga, even just yoga breathing, will calm you. Or you can go for a walk. Take a shower. Yell. Stomp your feet. Scream. Tell yourself, *I can do this*.

5. Place your hand over your heart. Breathe. Be okay with however you are in this moment.

6. If you're feeling overwhelmed with where you're at in your life, someone else has been there before. Make a conscious choice to reflect on the wisdom of others if you have not developed the ability to trust your own intuition.

CHAPTER 2

Getting on the Road

So, where was I? Oh yes, on my husband's jet, off to my treatment center to solve my *issues* and, in the words of my husband, *get fixed*. But right now, I had more important things on my mind.

For the duration of the flight, I worried over my daughters, who were fifteen and seventeen at the time. What had they been told, and how would my husband spin things? What were they thinking? Who would look out for them in my absence? Would they be all right?

Without doubt, my greatest life achievement has been bringing two wonderful girls into this world. My principle desire remains for their utmost happiness and well-being. Having them, however, was not an easy road.

Early in our marriage, I had a miscarriage without knowing I was pregnant. Only then did I start striving for a family; I guess I had assumed it would just happen. After trying for many years (five long years spent seeking out every infertility doctor and treatment known to man), we found out the "problem": my husband. As soon as they fixed him, I got pregnant.

It should have been the happiest time of my life, but two things happened in rapid succession. First, my insurance company cancelled my policy because I was "infertile." We had no money, and I think the stress of having a pregnant wife with no medical insurance broke my husband in some way. Second, when I had my first bout of morning sickness, and my ever-present smile and can-do attitude waned, my husband looked me right in the eyes and said, "Millions and millions of women have had children. Don't think you're doing anything special." I knew then that I had *serious* trouble.

But the last thing I wanted was a repeat of my childhood, this time me being the single mother, uneducated and struggling financially like my mother. At eighteen, I tried to put myself through school but had struggled to keep it all together, while holding down multiple jobs and a full course load. Several universities and countless wasted credits later, I finally quit. So, I dismissed his attack and focused on my quest to bear a healthy child. Because of his snide remark, I set out to prove to my husband and the world that I was neither flawed nor useless as a woman.

I ultimately had two beautiful, healthy girls, both of whom fill my heart with joy and completeness. I loved raising them and all those special solo times we shared. I often replay in my mind the memories of them playing at the park, sleepovers, soccer games, making pancakes, and driving them to piano lessons. I loved teaching them how to read, ride a bike, be kind to others, and pursue their passions.

I happily and often chose them over meeting with a client or my growing business. No one can take those years from me.

I consciously set an example I hoped would send my daughters out into the world as healthy women. I would tell them as I went off to the gym that I took care of myself so I could take care of them. In the world I modeled for them, women owned companies, played sports, and pursued their dreams. But somewhere along the way, our world—and my story—became distorted.

My daughters were home with my assistant when my husband returned from St. Barts on that fateful day. Exactly what they were told remains a mystery to me. It wouldn't surprise me if it sounded like something to the effect of, *Mommy is crazy and needs help*. How my situation was portrayed to them would later come to haunt me even to this day.

In his 2009 book, *A Promise to Ourselves: A Journey Through Fatherhood and Divorce*, American actor Alec Baldwin shone a spotlight on the damage of parental alienation—when one parent turns a child, or children, against the other parent. There's no doubt in my mind that my daughters have been emotionally damaged. Fortunately, I got out of my marriage and got help. My fear is that they won't get the help they still need to recover and heal.

I never viewed them as my property. I never sought approval and validation through the accomplishments of my daughters. It may seem odd to some parents, but I feel like pregnancy made me a vessel, gifted with the ability to give life to my daughters. I never felt that *they* were expressions of *my* worth.

They came into the world full of love and with special, unique personalities. I do believe I nurtured them as a loving mother; I also believe they have a lot of natural gifts I did *not* give them. A higher power gave them those.

You may be wondering what this has to do with me getting on the road of my own yoga journey. If you want to radically change your life, it's important to be inquisitive about how and why you are where you are at in your life. As well as decide that your situation could be different.

Once you've gotten specific about acting on your realization that you are going to change, there is only one requirement: a willingness to act.

Here's the good news: if you're open and willing, your actions will catalyze change.

As for me, I had a lot of work to do. I had to go back, way back to the beginning.

MY PARENTS

During what I would eventually call my midlife *adjustment*, I received a letter from my father, to whom I had not spoken for twenty-five years. I didn't open it for a week. The past, and the abuse I'd suffered at his hands, was the last thing I wanted to deal with in my then-present state.

I eventually opened my father's letter. He'd heard I was *going through something* and wanted to connect. The most compelling sentence? "I'm sorry I failed you as a father." Eight words on a page that would change his and my lives forever. I contacted him and decided to undertake the eleven-hour drive to his home in Colorado. I guess this would be remembered as my first Yoga Road Trip.

What do you say to someone after twenty-five years? The last time we'd spoken, I was newly engaged.

As a child, he petrified me. The worst part of the beatings was having to get the belt myself. Before striking me, he'd say, "This is going to hurt me more than it's going to hurt you." I wasn't even allowed to be the one in pain. As an eight-year old, following my parents' divorce, I blamed him for all the bad things in my (and my mom's and my brothers') life. I never gave him credit for anything good.

As I pulled into the driveway, he came out on the porch. "Hello, Stephanie. Welcome to Colorado." I said my fill. He said his. We made up. The little girl who still lives in me had a father again.

I learned that people do have the capacity to forgive and move forward. I still hold my father accountable for his actions. Do I blame him for everything bad in my life? No. Am I angry at times for having parents who clearly were either unprepared to have children or didn't want to? Sometimes. And I continue to work on that. My daughters, too, are victims of their parents' upbringing, and of generations of abuse on both sides of the family tree.

My father told me he's proud of me for having the courage to look at myself, work on myself, and grow. I'm proud of him, too. I value my time with him. Our conversations have been frank and open, two qualities I admire. I've learned from my father that I'm not going to *convince* my daughters, or anyone else for that matter, of my worth. I am who I am. He is who he is. Like all humans, we're flawed.

I recently learned that my father's been given a year to live. I know my time with him is limited. We have no regrets. We chose love.

My mother is another story. She denies any part in the abuse my two brothers and I suffered at our father's hands. She doesn't understand that because she didn't protect us, she is just as culpable. She should have left when it started, or at least sought help. But she feared him. *Like I did my husband. Before.*

Not only did she not leave, she threatened to kill herself every time my father said he wanted to get a divorce. This kept him, and the abuse, around longer. He finally left near my eighth birthday. And it stopped.

My mother, paranoid that I'd end up like her, then used fear to corrupt any healthy sense of self-esteem and sexuality I may have possessed. Because I grew up in this abusive and toxic family unit, confusion, fear, shame, and pain (both physical and emotional) were all I knew.

In treatment, I swirled in heartache with the knowledge that my daughters were destined to experience their own emotional pain.

SPIRITUAL WARRIOR WISDOM

Finding and practicing with inspiring yoga teachers have enhanced my life in deep and profound ways. They, too, gain from teaching and practicing with you. They are just like you. They move through the ups and downs of life in a graceful way because they practice yoga, and you will, too.

Stuck in my own crucible of despair, I could have escaped my own deception that life was just *going to be this way* had I found a trustworthy yoga teacher. Hanging out with a teacher like Jill Miller, because of my old back issues, would have been perfect physically. Emotionally, I had a lot to learn. Jill would have been an ideal source for inspiration.

Jill Miller

"I use the physical practice to minimize my stress and alter my reactivity. My emotions can get the better of me and sometimes cloud my ability to see the big picture.

My practice serves to give me critical distance from issues that I am troubled by or obsessing over. Often, I will have clarity, insight, and peace of mind about my next course of action after I practice.

Yoga has taught me to keep an open mind and to be acutely aware of my thoughts. It has given me tools to observe and change my reactivity. It has fostered a hunger to scrutinize my experience of embodiment that has led to thousands of hours of studies of anatomy, physiology, and movement sciences. It has helped me love life and choose positivity in spite of the range of complex and competing emotions that are a part of my daily journey."

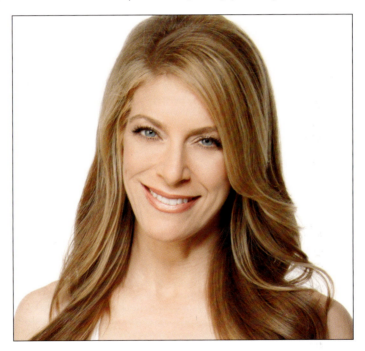

Practicing regularly with a raw, genuine, and caring soul like Jennica Mills would have launched me onto my new road much sooner. Suffering without self-awareness, I simply couldn't stay present to my experience. I'd simply checked out of my own life. It's called disassociation.

Jennica Mills

"In our society, we learn from an early age that our bodies are the enemy. We experience the body as we might an annoying little sibling that we can't get away from, can't seem to control, and who always seems to be a huge pain. Often, we want to change our bodies, or just simply pretend that they don't exist. This is due to a major lack of understanding of the body's basic functioning and innate intelligence.

The body has intuition. When I listen carefully and let go of control, I can heal, and experience freedom and connectedness. When I let my body move me, instead of me moving my body, I experience innate intelligence. Being gentle takes far more persistence and practice than pushing too hard. Being gentle cultivates the trust necessary to discover mastery.

The body responds the same way (in differing degrees) to a major trauma as it does to being fearful of a domineering boss or getting scolded by a teacher. Yogic practices help us to regulate the nervous system, bring homeostasis back to the body, and let go of old survival patterns that can make us physically ill and emotionally conflicted. Yoga allows us to be embodied once again and to cultivate a relationship with ourselves based on respect and curiosity. Maintaining presence allows you to thrive instead of just survive.

Yoga can be practiced anywhere at any moment. Most people imagine a serene, mat-lined room filled with superspiritual and/or incredibly flexible bodies moving into difficult postures. This is only one possibility in the infinite ways we can experience yoga.

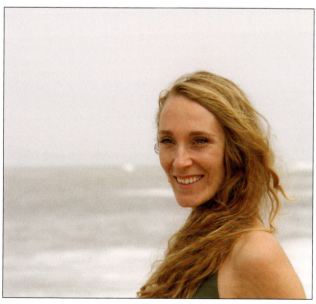

The science of yoga is so vast that it can effectively be used by simply becoming aware of the breath, sitting into one's current emotional state, feeding oneself a nourishing meal, chanting a healing mantra, praying, or giving the homeless person on the street your leftovers from dinner. Beyond the physical practice, yoga is a means of knowing oneself more deeply, loving oneself more fully, and connecting more authentically.

Practicing, you learn to embrace emotional states that you once deemed bad or negative as simply another human emotion on the continuum of what is possible. You can find joy and presence in sadness, anger, and grief. This human experience is nuanced and subtle.

I have personally used yoga to overcome my own challenges dealing with vicarious trauma and posttraumatic stress carried over from childhood. I use yoga to quiet my mind and get clarification about life challenges like relationship stress, major life changes, or low energy. Time and time again, I come back to the practice, and I am filled with hope. *Yoga has given me faith that I can overcome any challenge or ailment the body and mind can present."*

Jennica says, "isolation is an illusion." If you're feeling that you are alone right now, finish this chapter and find a respected yoga teacher near you. You should consult your physician or other healthcare professional before starting this or any other active exercise to determine if it is right for your needs. Certifications matter, so do your research. Many teachers have an online presence, and all those included in this book have a website. Most in this book have retreats all over the world. Yoga festivals are also an amazing way to take your practice to the next level. I love the energy of a live class. If you're new, go to a beginner's class. Introduce yourself to the teacher.

Teachers lovingly want to be there for you. Get to know yours. They will be there for you. Tanya Markul was there when I was ready to change my life. She teaches and writes about courageous authenticity. Her writing speaks to millions around the world. If you can, commit to becoming a student for life. Imagine how you could love being a student of your life.

Tanya Markul

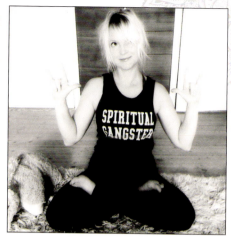

"The most important ingredient you can put into anything is you.

This is our time, and there is so much to be done. This moment is the perfect time to re-evaluate who and what we think we are and to start 'doing' in the direction of our hearts. We've been manipulated to hide our abilities, to be fearful of nature, to shun our magic, to not question the things we know deep down inside aren't right, leading us to believe that our life experience is hopeless, that change is not possible. It's time to remove this veil and to allow us to be empowered by a self-worth that is nourishing from the inside out. It's time to delicately use darkness as it was meant to be used—as an indicator of light, deep wisdom, healing, and limitless imagination.

Creativity is what we are—every single person on this planet has a creative ability. No one can tell *your* story like *you* can, and we're creating this story every single day with our voices, our eyes, our hands, our mindsets, our bodies. We were born into certain situations, and it is that warriorship that is ours to define, redefine, and create to the best of our own personal ability. The question is—Can we evolve from it? Can we live deeply without force and without trying to control everyone and everything? Can we give love and, more important, can we receive it? And can we find and become our authentic selves in this lifetime?

These sentiments are essences of yoga. *Yoga invites us into an intimate inquiry of ourselves by creating a dialogue between the mind, body, and spirit.* The practice draws us toward scary edges, and, sooner or later, layers upon layers start to unfold, reconstruct, open, and heal. An awakening happens. This is a beautiful creative process, and, more than anything, it's individual. The experience of yoga is yours to discover.

Yoga has taught me to feel and follow the intuition of my body—with awareness, sensitivity, and honesty. Just a little bit more mindfulness in every single human being could significantly change the course of life for all life forms on the planet today. Mix that with a bit of unrelenting tenderness, gentle truths, less control, and fear, and we may just end up with heaven on earth."

Realize that you're powerful. One of the best things about my life challenge was this: I figured out that the best way to nourish myself is by surrounding myself with amazing people like Tanya, and teachers like MacKenzie Miller. MacKenzie's words are like a trusted pep talk. It's like when your best friend and you call each other at the same time. You know you're not alone. If you've ever known what it's like to be lonely, I can guarantee you there are people who would love to connect with you. Get to a yoga class. Say hello to someone.

MacKenzie Miller

"Yoga has taught me how capable I am of achieving anything I put my mind to.

Yoga is for everyone. It is now. Don't wait for the right moment, flexibility, or whatever excuse you're using. The practice is healing and ready to embrace you if you're ready to embrace it. Find the right type of yoga for you, which means you try different types and instructors until you find what works. Once you do, you'll gift yourself the power to change your life.

Yoga is how I've overcome all the hardships throughout my life. As a child, I wasn't given the tools to healthily deal with strong emotions, and through a long series of losses, I created a thick skin from numbing the pain that was never dealt with. Thanks to my yoga practice, I have worked through that and continue to work on my issues. Yoga has opened my heart to accepting my humanity and being vulnerable enough to ask for help when needed. There have been some

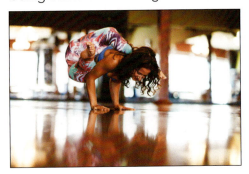

dark periods in my life, but now when life gets messy, my yoga practice carries me through. I no longer turn to numbing substances or any other self-destructive mechanisms. I meditate. Every day I give thanks for my yoga practice.

My mantra is frequently *I am enough*. The beauty of that statement is, it rings true for you, too."

I continue to use the mantra *I am enough* in times of insecurity. I'm grateful to know MacKenzie. I'm glad you now do, too. Being whole is being balanced. Balance means equal proportions. Sri Dharma Mittra is equal parts wise, authentic, and caring. Teachers exist to help you become your best once you have become a willing participant. Great teachers are warm, enthusiastic, and accessible.

Sri Dharma Mittra is just that kind of person: inviting, knowledgeable, and grounded. Don't be intimidated by people who teach at big yoga conferences. Search for a teacher who resonates with your needs, even one who challenges you. Flying off into the unknown, I needed a kick in the you-know-what.

Sri Dharma Mittra

"Yoga taught me all about my personal self (the non-self, the mind), and also, the true cause of pain and delusion. I have learned lots of techniques to remove the obstacles on the way to self-realization. My compassion was upgraded to go beyond my relatives, friends and pets—to learn to see myself in others. With some success along the way, I realized that the purpose of life is to help others and to achieve self-realization, liberation, or enlightenment.

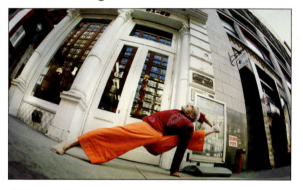

It was more than fifty years ago when it happened. At that time, I had lots of doubts, delusion, and pain. I read a book about yoga. It was about self-knowledge, mental powers, and Samadhi. I was fascinated with it, and, with all my heart, I believed in what it had to say, especially with regard to reincarnation, the laws of karma, self-realization, and the states of bliss after enlightenment. As a result of reading this book, I immediately made the divine decision to seek yoga instruction. In 1964, I met my teacher, and that was it! I really got hooked on yoga and, of course, on him (my Guru), too. Soon after meeting my teacher, I made the decision to become a full-time yogi.

See yourself in others. This must reach beyond your relatives, friends, and pets. If everyone understood this, how in the world could, or would, anyone hurt anyone else? This is a very efficient way for you to instantly upgrade your compassion. With compassion, one gets a little bit more spiritually civilized. With the ability to place ourselves in others, it's the first step to self-realization. This makes us more respectful, reverent, and compassionate to all. As a result, we gain peace of mind and freedom from delusion.

With all the wisdom of yoga—that's to say, the results of constant yoga practice—the realization of lots of sacred knowledge, some self-control, and armed with full compassion, an amazing spiritual enthusiasm is always present and, thus, you can easily overcome any challenge—I mean all of them!"

Hearing others share that they, too, had "doubts, delusion, and pain" has been a huge gift. Many of the teachers in this book are successful, published authors. Their books can help you as well if you are unable to ever physically take a class with them. Smile in the understanding that reading is a powerful way to grow. People who read are smart. The trick is to apply the wisdom.

Teachers understand your challenges because they have them, too. The difference between balanced, healthy people and unbalanced people is priorities. Make yourself your priority. Get specific about getting on the road. As Honza and Claudine Lafond explain, "in every breath there is an opportunity for transformation." At the time of my crash, I was stuck: personal transformation was the furthest idea from my mind.

Honza and Claudine both exist in a supportive and healthy space as a couple. That concept in a relationship was foreign to me back then. As you can clearly see in the visually stunning images they share online, they also physically support each other in Acrovinyasa yoga. They appear together in many poses, but they also teach numerous forms of yoga movement and self-expression. They introduced me to what it could look like to have the same value set as a couple. What they teach, and live, is wellness.

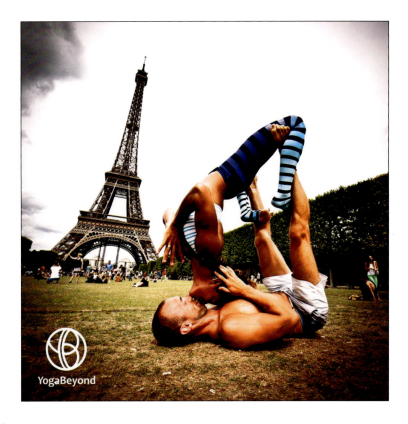

HEALING THE HEART, SOUL, AND BODY

Honza Lafond

"Yoga has taught me to be patient. It has instilled a deeper understanding of my reactions and actions to every situation, and for that, I have become a changed human being. It has taught me so much about the connection to my breath. I have come to realize that Pranayama is a powerful tool that has expanded my life in so many ways. *In every breath lies another opportunity to tune in to the present moment.*"

Claudine Lafond

"Yoga has taught me that there is so much more than my physical body. My journey started when I was just beginning to ask myself the larger questions of my life purpose and what it all means. I often say, as many others have also claimed, that yoga saved my life. Once I discovered the good medicine in yoga, and realized that everything I needed to heal, transform, and live a blissful life was already within, I felt at peace. I recognized that we are all lifelong students.

My yoga journey began at the age of fifteen in Bali. I was invited to an Iyengar Yoga class in a beautiful garden at someone's home. We practiced in an outdoor gazebo with birds chirping and cows grazing nearby. At the end of the practice, we all sat around drinking chai and talking (well, I was just listening) yoga philosophy. I went back every day for the next five weeks. I was hooked.

At the time I started teaching, I simply loved to connect with other people and have a shared experience of movement. I felt that if just one person had a shift in class, that was good enough for me. I still feel grounded and humble but realize that the ripple effect now is very powerful.

Yoga isn't a practice limited to a mat, nor is it a practice available only to a certain group of people. It is a powerful tool for transformation and healing and should be available to everybody in the world. It is not just about physical postures and breathing. This is just the tip of the iceberg. *Yoga is an outlook on life and a state of being.* You'll never know what yoga is all about unless you give it a try."

I can relate to Honza and Claudine's desire to spread the message of yoga to as many people as possible. The yoga community includes many unique voices. What is similar is the love, kindness, and care teachers bring to it. They will show you the way yoga can help you cultivate the things you need to create mindfulness and self-discovery. They are deeply committed to your growth.

Like all learning, it takes practice. Consider saying to yourself, "I'm doing the best that I can."

Once I got on the road, I started to unravel the abuse in my life. One of the people I met who had a huge impact on my life, and continues to do so, is Rolf Gates. When I first heard about Rolf, I was told that I would relate to his story. Uncertain how, I picked up his best-selling book, **Meditations from the Mat**, and could not put it down. I knew I had to meet him. When I did, I was struck by his gentle, brilliant, and passionate soul. He is so genuine and real. There's no faster way to get real than to get honest with yourself. I was ready.

Rolf Gates

"I came into my spiritual practice through recovery from addiction. The first things I got in rehab were these 24-hour books, and it really helped to have something that was small. My attention span was short at the time. Everyone would read and talk about them. That was a big part of developing a spiritual practice in that world.

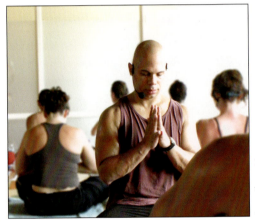

I've always been able to be consistent in all that I do. I need things that get me excited about what I am doing. I try to get into the spirit of things. Whatever I get into, I like to get into the joy of it.

There are so many great teachers in my life. Marianne Williamson, Deepak Chopra, and people like that. I read a lot. Spiritual means, to me, that what you are reading today is going to be applied to your life today. You need to be reminded of humility or generosity, or reminded that the path goes forward, then back. And then you go out and apply it.

When I got into yoga, it surprised me that there was no easy vehicle to learn about the yoga sutras. At the time, you had to plow through a huge academic tome to learn about it, and no one was into that. Everyone else just didn't know what yoga was. The people I met were taking yoga at a gym. They liked 'yoga,' but they didn't really understand it.

I believe that, if people can understand what yoga is, they can make good choices for themselves about how to develop their practice. I remain motivated to spreading the word about what yoga really is."

I'm honored that Rolf believed in me and my project. He was on board from the get-go. Once you identify mentors in your life, they step up to support you. I'm sure Christina Sell can point to her yoga mentors, having come to the practice so young.

Christina Sell

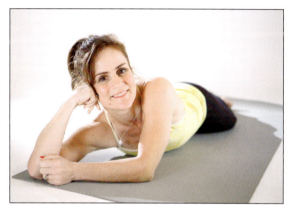

"I got started on my yoga journey when I was eighteen. I went to treatment for bulimia and depression. I spent eighteen months in a residential program, where I was introduced to twelve-step recovery, cathartic emotional work, and a path of rigorous self-honesty that included many practical tools for introspection and self-inquiry.

Yoga asana wasn't love at first sight or in any way dramatic for me. I felt good after class, I enjoyed learning the postures, and I loved the mindful rigor of the Iyengar Yoga style of practice.

Yoga is not only asana practice. *Yoga is all the tools, techniques, and practices that comprise a spiritual path.* Some of those tools and techniques are outer practices, like asana, meditation, or mantra. Some of the tools are internal and involve awareness, attention, intention, and remembrance. The inner tools can be brought to bear on every life circumstance so that a fusion between yoga and life occurs where life becomes yoga in a practical and immediate way.

Yoga and life are not different things, and each one informs the other. I believe that life is perfectly designed to produce the experiences, lessons, challenges, and insights I need to evolve spiritually, and the practices are about helping me make use of what my life is providing me all the time.

Yoga is definitely not for those people who do not want to change or who do not want to apply themselves to the process of growth. Yoga does not exist separately from the practitioner. If you like devotional practices, you should do them. If you like more athletic endeavors, do them. There is a lot of 'noise' out there about what yoga is and the right way to practice and the wrong way to practice. The best practice is the one that you do, and the one you will stick with is the one that you enjoy."

By being inquisitive about yourself, as Christina is, you have the perfect opportunity to grow. You don't have to do it alone.

If you need help, ask for it. Once you acknowledge that, your life will never be the same, because admitting your truth creates momentum. I had to accept that I wasn't even in the car on the ride of my life. By being curious about how and why you are wanting to change, an on-ramp will appear.

HERE'S WHAT I LEARNED ABOUT GETTING ON THE ROAD:

1. You may need help. I don't believe we are meant to travel alone on our path to awakening. Get professional help if you need it. Find a yoga teacher. Tell them why you are there. Have the courage to ask for what you need.

2. Once you're awake (on the road), there's no turning around. That's a good thing, trust me.

3. There will be potholes, detours, and a flat tire or two. When you finally get a patch of smooth pavement, it's time to accelerate your efforts.

4. I recognized that the tools I'd relied upon had created a strong, resilient, and brave person. Stop and acknowledge the gifts of growth. Self-awareness through the work that you are doing, on and off your mat, is extremely valuable. You're going to rely on these to stay on your road.

CHAPTER 3

Reading Your Life Road Map

After touching down in the beautiful Arizona desert, the limo in which my therapist and I were traveling passed a famous spa I'd been to almost a dozen times. I knew this spa well because I had escorted readers of my wellness magazine there for years. As we drove past, I contemplated the time I had spent working there. I knew this had to be very different from the work I had done at a spa. Nervous? You bet, but engaged. I didn't discuss my thoughts with the therapist. I had hardly spoken to her the whole trip.

OFF TO TREATMENT CENTER ONE (TC1)

I didn't know how badly I needed to get out of my environment. I needed space to focus on me and my issues, to free myself from the trauma and abuse that had consumed so much of my life. To understand why I had allowed myself to be a passenger in someone else's car wreck.

Fear of my life remaining the same motivated me to go, but I also dwelled in fear of what would happen if I didn't agree to go.

We arrived at a complex that looked quite like the spa we had just passed, complete with Spanish architecture and lush desert surroundings, innocently imagining that this wasn't going to be as bad as I feared. Once inside, the center looked more like a hospital with a dash of nursing home décor. We walked up to reception, I signed myself in, and my therapist and I parted ways. Finally, I was on my own.

The escort took me down a long, stark hallway to a dorm-like room resembling one found in an orphanage, full of small beds. Next, the kind soul led me into a meeting room, where I took my seat in the circle and, one by one, we introduced ourselves and shared why we were there. Crack. Heroin. Alcohol. Cocaine. I chimed in, "Ambien," and everyone laughed.

One of the therapists leading the session motioned for me to leave with her, then led me into a small office with a metal desk and two chairs. She gave me a sheet of paper with a list of terms, each with an adjacent tick box. This person, whom I would never see again, asked me to check any boxes with terms with which I could identify that I had experienced at some point in my lifetime. The list included things like receiving beatings, emotional manipulation, bullying, intimidation, objectification as a sexual object, painful or unwanted touch, denial of medical care, negative self-talk, and ignoring my own needs. *I checked every box on the page.*

Immediately, they moved me out of the Addiction program and into the Trauma and Abuse wing. You may be thinking, *I can't relate to this heavy stuff. I'm just trying to lose a couple of pounds or live with less stress.*

Before you can change, you need to unfreeze. Think of it like pulling something out of the freezer to thaw before you cook it. Because many people will naturally resist change, the goal at this fork in the road is to create an awareness of how the status quo is hindering your ability to live in balance. If you were already living at your highest potential, you may not have picked up this book.

Awareness must be carefully examined to understand how necessary a change is, as well as the logic behind it. The more you know about why you need to change, and feel that it is necessary and urgent, the more motivated you are to accept the change.

The next morning, I sat in a huge circle alongside hundreds of patients. We each introduced ourselves with labels such as "codependent," "mood disorder," "addict," and our choice of nine declarative words describing how we were feeling: "happy," "sad," "tired," etc. It was surreal.

Surrounding me were people in various stages of pain, people who'd been abused, neglected, and traumatized, many of them victims of parents who never should have had children. As a writer, I'd always had an insatiable appetite for *other* people's stories; I see now that I didn't realize I had a *story of my own.*

During my first daily two-hour group therapy session, which included six patients and two therapists, I listened in shock as my comrades described how and why they'd tried to kill themselves. My mind raced with thoughts of, *I'm in the wrong group!* or, *Holy shit, do they think I belong here?* Looking back, I feel sorry for the scared little girl sitting in that chair, who looks about seven or eight, staring in disbelief at what is happening around her. She has no voice, no ability to express what she thinks, and is so gripped by terror that no words will come out. I know that girl now; I didn't know her then.

We were given a writing assignment: to compose a description of ourselves. What immediately popped into my head? A vision of a Lonely Warrior, wearing armor and riding a horse. Life, to me, had always been a battle: a battle for emotional, physical, and spiritual survival. Very *Joan of Arc*, dirty and deter-mined, yet ineffective. As I wrote about the Lonely Warrior, the Rolling Stones' song "I Can't Get No Satisfaction" played in my head.

Since I could remember, I'd always been striving and doing, driven by an in-satiable quest for perfection, yet ineffective in accomplishing the things I really wanted. The ponytailed Lonely Warrior was now exhausted from years of fight-ing, with a smile plastered on the beautiful mask she wore to disguise her pain.

I was given the opportunity to unravel the ties dragging me into the apathetic pit of the world I inhabited. I'd bought into the idea that it was best to just swirl around in someone else's tornado, drama, and crazymaking. I was such a part of my husband's world that his tornado had become a part of mine. At the Center, I realized, I could learn to reconnect with my strength, resiliency, and courage, the very things that had enabled me to survive the traumas I'd endured, some of which I'd erased from my memory.

During a Psychodrama session, we were reenacting the events of another patient's past in which a motorcycle gang held her captive for a week. Psychodrama is a form of psychotherapy in which participants act out traumatic events from their past. It is often used as a psychotherapy, in which clients use spontaneous dramatization, role playing, and dramatic self-presentation to in-vestigate and gain insights into their lives. Yes, I know this all sounds dark and heavy, and it was. During the session, we each reenacted her torture, rape, and humiliation, in turn, pretending to cut her with blades, blindfold her, strap her to a chair, and beat her with boards as she wept. *It felt like new trauma to me.*

A week later, during a treatment called Eye Movement Desensitization and Reprocessing (EMDR), I unlocked an old secret I'd buried deep inside. At the age of fifteen, I'd been gang-raped at a friend's pool party in Houston. Even now, my only memory is of my friend's older brother on top of me, crying, "Oh God, there's blood!" He'd stolen my virginity. I remember another *friend* being invited to climb on top of me because he too had never done *it* before. I recall one other form on top of me, but can't see his face. I don't know if they gave me a date-rape drug, or if my memory of the event is still deeply repressed, despite the unraveling I've done.

After a month, I left the treatment center. I'd "fixed" my Ambien dependency. I was ready to get my divorce. I was excited to create a new life, to embrace a whole new beginning. Most important, to reunite with my daughters, whom I'd missed terribly. I wanted us together and wanted to hear from them and under-stand their feelings, positive or negative, about what was happening. What I wanted was an entirely new relationship dynamic with them.

However, my treatment center therapist suggested, and I agreed, that I should not go home yet. While I had changed, radically, he reminded me that home remained the same environment, the same people—a place where nothing had changed. So, I followed the advice to work on *reentry* at another treatment center in New Mexico before returning to Pittsburgh.

SPIRITUAL WARRIOR WISDOM

There's no faster way to improve your life than to tune in to accountability. You can't fix what you don't know is broken.

I needed to change my life, and I had committed to understanding why. At the treatment center, I felt like I had been handed a magnifying glass to the road map of my life. Upon examination, I could see what had possibly been hiding in my rearview mirror, around the corner on a dangerous road. Sounds complicated? Heck yeah.

We're amazingly complex creatures. We're also divinely simple, if given a chance to see that. Yoga can give you the gift of the ability to see yourself for who you are. To look inward. To grow. Which brings me to another *growth facilitator*, Adri Kyser. Adri reminds me that no matter where you are on your yoga journey, you can always go deeper. Although I had been practicing for years, at the time of my crash, I still had much to learn. For Adri, transforming her personal practice took focus and the courage to examine deeply her inner self. Something I had yet to undertake.

Adri Kyser

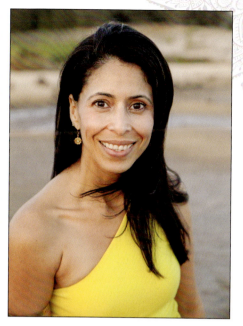

"Yoga helped me go within and heal aspects of myself that I was not aware of. It has helped me find my voice and purpose. Yoga has inspired me to follow my dreams, to love and respect myself, and it has deepened my connection to God, The Universe, The Divine Spirit.

Everyone, regardless of age, gender, belief, size, or shape, can practice yoga. Yoga is not a religion or a sequence of extreme poses. *Yoga is a way of self-(re) discovery and connection to the Source. It is both the way and the tool that brings us back to a state of wholeness and well-being.* Yoga has become my refuge in moments of despair.

It has been my companion in moments of difficulty. Even when I don't want to step on my mat, I find that my practice can consist of a variety of (or just a single) simple gestures or actions, like lighting a candle and sitting in silence, or journaling, breathing consciously, or praying.

My personal yoga practice has transformed from being mainly asana-based to many forms of connectivity, trust, devotion, and surrender."

Smile with the understanding that you have the ultimate champion in your corner. It's you. You simply need to look with new eyes. It's like seeing yourself in the mirror after a long hot shower and recognizing that your face has changed since the last time you studied your reflection. See yourself beyond the physical appearance. Strive to remove the tendency to assign a positive or negative definition to what you see. Instead, look deep into your reflection at how perfect you are, flaws and all. Have gratitude that you are seeking a better version of you.

By being inquisitive about evaluating your reflection and your life road map, you move forward in your growth—on your yoga path to self-transformation. Never has this been more succinctly said than by Gary Chattem, a fixture in my online community. I added Gary to my online community because of his inspiring feed.

Gary Chattem

"Yoga taught me that almost anything is possible. We have a lot more self-determination in creating our reality than we give ourselves credit for.

Yoga is for everyone. You don't need to go to a studio. Use a Vedic chart to determine what yoga is best for you. I started Bikram for healing. Yoga IS the prescription. That is where my healing came from."

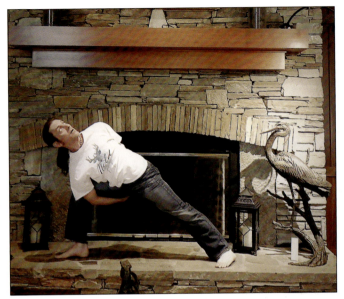

Your reality is created through your senses. Your online experience either adds to or detracts from your reality. Drown yourself in the sea of knowledge and inspiration that is online. Use social media and the Internet to enhance your day, just like I did by selecting positive online friends like Gary. Your time online is either taking you down the right road or an unhealthy one. Use discernment to eliminate toxic words, people, and images from your view.

Carve out time in your day to shut off your smartphone, close your eyes, and simply focus on your breath for five minutes. If you're unable to make it through the day without being wired, use your tools to elevate your life instead of distracting you from yourself. There are many online resources, especially on YouTube. For example, videos on cardiac coherence, where you watch, say, a water drop go up and down and breathe in sync with it.

Intimately sharing with brave and authentic people who could have inspired me would have been priceless. Jacoby Ballard is just such a person, a survivor of childhood sexual abuse who faced his abusers. Knowing him, perhaps I could have understood the need to acknowledge and deal with the realities of my own abuse.

Jacoby Ballard

"I have come out as queer, as trans, and as a survivor of childhood sexual abuse through my practice. I have confronted both blood family and chosen family patterns of addiction through my practice.

My practice has taught me what my life's dharma, or purpose, is. Every day before I meditate, I read my purpose aloud, recentering and remembering why I am living each day. *Yoga has allowed me to slow down, be still, and examine, rather than just constantly be in motion, a pattern from being both a survivor and part of a marginalized community.* Constant movement because the present is so painful and overwhelming if one doesn't have the skills and community to be with it. Yoga has turned me back toward what I might otherwise run from due to various forms of trauma. Through compassion, patience, presence, forgiveness, and Beginner's Mind, I come back to those situations and people that remind me of my trauma.

Perhaps most important, yoga has taught me about interdependence and connection, and that I need my teachers and community . . . the same way my students need me. Yoga and Buddhism have taught me gratitude for this circle

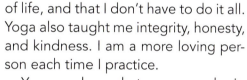
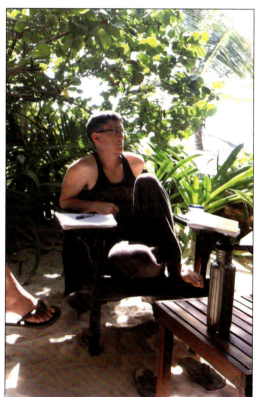

of life, and that I don't have to do it all. Yoga also taught me integrity, honesty, and kindness. I am a more loving person each time I practice.

Yoga makes whatever you do in your life better, be it lifting weights, being a parent, making music, creating pottery, designing a building, whatever . . . because it enables you to shed layers of expectation, pressure, and trauma so you can come to your truth and let your work emerge from a place of love.

Yoga adds magic to what you do and accentuates what makes your life worth living. It is not about having a flexible body, but a flexible mind and heart. But when you shed layers of tension from your body, you do so from your mind/heart as well, which is why the physical practice is important. Yoga is also just one wisdom tradition, one peel of the banana. There are many other approaches, so the key to accessing this magic is to find the modality or spirituality that makes your life sparkle and shine.

I just come to my mat, and my cushion, again and again, and listen. I bring my whole self, my anger, my joy, my jealousy, my grief, my pain, my tears, my laughter, and work with the energy. I have learned to be exactly what I need in that moment.

Yoga also has challenges within it. Read a teacher's bio before entering their classroom. The energy of so many studios is about competition, ascent, and individualism, and I choose not to put myself in those kinds of environments anymore. Through my practice, I realize that I have a choice to not put myself in harm's way when I see it coming. I have been incredibly injured as a queer and trans person in the yoga classroom. I could run screaming from that situation and never enter a studio again and have made that choice at moments. But my practice is to come back to yoga communities and be in the pain of transphobia, homophobia, racism, ableism, fat phobia, and allow my experience with that pain to expand my heart. And to teach others that the extent to which I feel pain, I feel joy, as well—the heart expands in both directions.

In coming out as trans and identifying along the masculine spectrum, it has been rewarding for me to have influence on men around oftentimes challenging topics including sexism, misogyny, and patriarchy. I was abused by boys, threatened all my life as a girl by men, and am the child of a second-wave feminist who constantly spoke to microaggressions that men perpetuate. Masculine-presenting people have such privilege in our society, even within our queer communities, and women and feminine-presenting people daily face such violence, I believe that it is our duty as men to challenge violent forms of masculinity, out of our love for all of humanity, and to cultivate the courage to embrace our own femininity, as well. Coming out as trans has also allowed me to embrace my femininity too, so I do this work to create more space for myself, and every other human being."

As inspiring and uplifting as Jacoby is for stepping into the light, I was a fearful soul hiding behind a mask, hiding in the dark. A strong way to step into the light is to acknowledge that you're not in a great place. Kate Kendall told me that yoga helped give her fearless self-inquiry to begin again on a journey of a life she had never imagined.

Kate Kendall

"Do not take life too seriously, your body is your greatest tool for decision making (so look after it!), and the only thing that's constant is change."

We can practice yoga anywhere. I know yogis who have never taken a physical posture or asana in their lives, but they're yogis because they understand the concept of presence, they do things wholeheartedly, and they attract positive people and situations because they're aware of their connection to self and everyone else.

When I got into yoga, I wasn't in a great place, mentally. In my teens, I was diagnosed with anorexia, and even though I recovered physically quite quickly, mentally, I took a while longer and spiraled into depression and was eventually put on antidepressants. After my year-long party in London, yoga was that thing that was meant to 'tone' my body again. Little did I know that, one month after practicing yoga four times a week consistently, I would be off my meds and journeying into a life I never imagined.

Yoga has taught me to self-inquire fearlessly. Yoga has also taught me that we're part of a bigger picture, and we're all in this magnificent masterpiece together. When we work together, give to one another, and practice compassion, life's that much more vibrant and juicy.

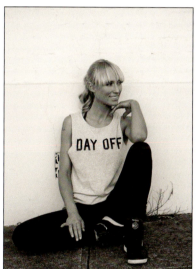

Part of depression, for me, was feeling disconnected. So, at my studio, we have managed to create a community of yogis and 'athletes' who vibe off one another in class, connect, and make friends. Knowing that we're connecting people is what it's all about. It makes a huge difference.

It's about doing one thing at a time, and with your whole heart. It's about tasting life, savoring and enjoying the small things that we forget with the rush of life."

Before I could go deeper, I needed time to examine whether I was the passenger or the driver in my car of life. Whatever brings you to yoga, know that it's at the perfect time, just as it was for Kate. Yulady Saluti started yoga to find hope and to deal with illness. Through the process of yoga, she discovered herself, and how we all can live in the moment.

Yulady Saluti

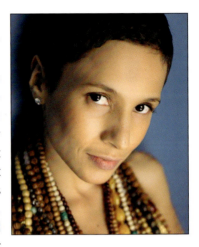

"During my illness, and fighting chronic pain and discomfort, my husband suggested I change my diet and start to exercise.

Yoga has introduced me to myself. Yoga has allowed me to see past my own problems, to see past the 'story' my ego created for me, making me a *sick person*. Yoga has helped me to tame my ego and see my true self, full of joy and passion. It has also allowed me to learn to live in the present moment. For a long time, I dwelled on my various illnesses. However, the life lessons I have learned, and continue to learn, from yoga both amaze and astound me every day. There really is nothing but the present moment, and by the way, that moment is perfect. My suffering invariably comes from thinking about the past or the future. Learn to live in the present moment, and life is a simple joy.

The physical benefits of yoga cannot be denied. If you practice asana, you will feel better and be healthier. The true poetry of yoga comes when the physical practice is transcended and you learn how the movement and breath, once connected, become a graceful dance and balance of ultimate presence and meditation.

Yoga helps you overcome challenges by allowing you to see the challenge as an opportunity to grow.

Everything that life presents to you is an opportunity. What you do with the opportunity will define your life. Yoga allows me to see what is truly important, like my husband, children, and friends, and what is not, like material things, being popular, and excess in general. Yoga has opened my eyes to the infinite possibilities the Universe has to offer us. I now see inspiration and beauty in places I would have never even thought to look, like a simple cloud in the sky or flower in the Earth. These are the things that yoga has given me."

It isn't always easy to see how a challenge can be anything but awful. The inspiration from witnessing Yulady move through her life with grace is like watching yoga work its infinite miracle daily. Even in the midst of a huge life shift, a huge challenge, I knew that defining a new journey was critical to recalibrating my life. The grace Richard Miller brings to the ongoing global yoga conversation continues to show me I was reaching out to and embracing a healthy new circle of contemporaries.

Richard Miller

"The practices and perspective of yoga have revealed that I am a unique, yet inseparable, expression of life, interconnected with all beings, animate and inanimate, everywhere. Knowing this has awakened deep love and compassion within me and propelled me into a life of service.

The underlying principle of yoga, for me, is welcoming, whereby I've learned to listen to, accept, welcome, and respond to each sensation, feeling, emotion, thought, and experience that comes my way. Because yoga has revealed my nonseparation with all of life, it's shown me that I contain within myself the perfect response to each moment that life brings to my table. As I welcome each moment, I can sense the response that's perfect for each situation, and in harmony with all of life."

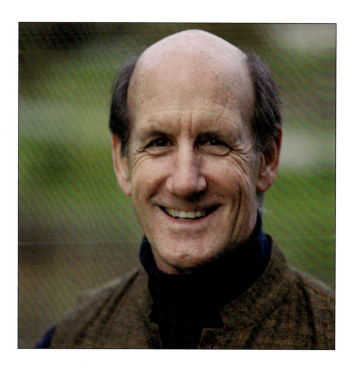

Connecting with incredible yoga teachers who are also authors kept me on the right path. Teachers like Carol Horton, who showed me that becoming "more meaningfully connected to others" was critical for charting and navigating a new path.

Carol Horton

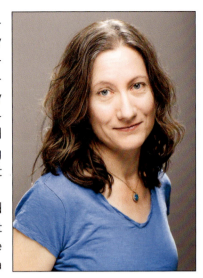

"Yoga has taught me that I have the power to connect to deeper parts of my own being on a daily basis, and that doing so enriches my life immeasurably. It has also taught me that my own self-development as a human being is inextricably linked to the process of becoming more meaningfully connected to others and the world around me. Daily practice helps me to trust that taking action to manifest what I intuitively feel is most meaningful is indeed a worthwhile endeavor.

For me, the path of yoga is not easy. I've asked myself whether I'm crazy to care so much about it more times than I could possibly count. Yet I've consistently found that yoga works for me on a deep level. Slacking off on my practice negatively impacts my health and happiness—and, since I prefer to be healthy and happy, I keep going back. I'm very grateful to have learned how to practice yoga.

Popular media images of yoga have caused lots of people to think that you need to be thin, fit, and flexible to do it. That's not true. Really, you simply need to be conscious—that is, not asleep, in a coma, intoxicated, or otherwise incapacitated. Yoga is the integration of mind, movement, and breath. Being able to focus your attention fully on your breath and bodily sensations for even a minute is much more 'yogic' than executing a gymnastic pose while your mind is racing and distracted.

Yoga is about internal experience, not physical prowess. It works with the body as a means of deepening and expending consciousness, not as an end in itself.

Yoga strengthens my ability to stay present with difficult emotions, feelings, and sensations and lessen my reactivity to them. The more I can live with the awareness that I'm experiencing fear, sadness, anger, or some other challenging state without immediately needing to act out, distract myself, or otherwise try to escape it, the more I can gain insight into it and enable myself to process in ways that support growth."

As with any new thing you're learning, be kind to yourself. As an engaged participant, you will tap into your "own potential and strength," as Kristin McGee knows and shares.

Kristin McGee

"Yoga has taught me to be more compassionate to myself and others. Yoga reminds me that life is a process. Through yoga, I've learned to go with the flow. I've discovered how to open myself up, physically and mentally, to new experiences.

Yoga has taught me how to tap in to my own potential and strength. Yoga has given me flexibility and helped me bounce back if I fall. Most important, I've learned that life really is the most amazing when I'm truly in the moment and cherishing each breath I take.

I tap into my breathing and go back to the basics of what's most important in life. I know that if I can hold myself up and support myself physically in yoga, I can do the same in life.

Yoga has taught me how to trust myself, that when I fall, I can pick myself back up and get back into position. I try and carry what I've learned on the mat into my life."

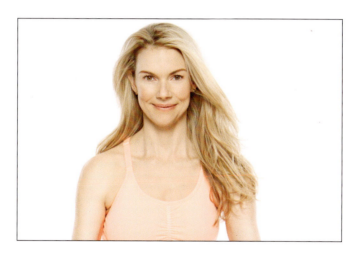

Kristin, just like you and me, encounters adversities big and small on and off her mat every day. It's your choice how to respond to those adversities that defines your life. Your moments. Yoga had to become something much more than a physical practice for me to overcome mine. I didn't need a physical life shift as much as an emotional and spiritual transformation.

I reached out to Ashley Turner, because she had long since moved past the physical benefits of yoga and was infusing her teachings with yoga psychology and philosophy.

Ashley Turner

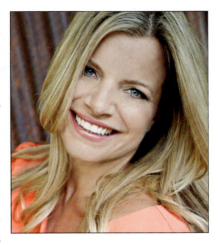

"I think yoga has taught me to identify more with my soul and more with my soul's journey than the physical reality of life and all of the external trappings, which are always falling and rising and changing forms around us.

So, it really keeps me tethered to a larger conversation, and enables me to keep asking different questions. When things are happening, when the shit is going down, how to ask different questions like 'What am I learning from this? How is this healing for me?' Moving from judgment to understanding. And the same is true with life: focusing on the process rather than on the outcome or any particulars.

I try to look at anything that arises and soften, physically and mentally. I try and be present with any emotions, feelings, and thoughts.

We—our mind and our ego, our society—are very tempted to focus and value our experience and ourselves based on all these external barometers, and none of those really matter. We all want the same thing: to love and be loved. So, how loving can you be?

How loving can you be with yourself? How much can you love other people? How much can you fall in love with your fate? How loving can you be with other people?

And, at the same time, be doing what you can to expand your awareness and your consciousness. And every day, doing practices that keep you wakeful and mindful, and showing up with the strongest, clearest, most balanced energy.

And with that being said, we're human. So, really allowing ourselves to be human, and practicing massive self-compassion and radical self-acceptance, really and truly softening our perceptions.

And being much more kind in every way. To ourselves. To one another. To life itself."

Extending kindness to yourself was a skill I had yet to fully understand. Lacking in self-awareness, I needed new tools in my toolkit. I'm a huge fan of the growing world of podcasts. They are a go-to tool for me, especially J. Brown's *Yoga Talk*. He has first-hand experience using yoga to enable him to process an experience within a relationship.

J. Brown

"My mother died of leukemia when I was sixteen years old.

In the years that followed, disillusionment set in gradually. At some point, I got very low, so low that I felt I either needed to kill myself or find another way to live. Fortunately, I chose the latter.

The course of my yoga practice has been the process of reconciling with my mother's death. It's difficult to explain how doing breathing and moving exercises can, inadvertently, carry with them the weight of facing mortality. Something about bringing careful attention to my breath and body, the most tangible expression of the fact that I am currently alive and the very thing that will be taken away from me in death, provides an experience that lessens the burdens I carry and illuminate's life's inherent worth.

From this standpoint, overcoming the difficulties that life presents becomes a celebratory endeavor, and I feel strangely grateful for my mother's passing. The pain and sorrow I feel because of my mother's death, still just as powerful today as when I was sixteen years old, are what led me to yoga and a deeper appreciation for life's blessings. My life has a deeper sense of purpose as a result. Yoga is not hard.

Setting aside the overarching philosophical frameworks at work, the conventional attitude is that to progress in practice, it is necessary to take your body past your perceived physical edge. Not taking your body past its physical edge is often seen as lazy or resistant. The practice is a way to challenge ourselves to do more, to reach fuller potential. And certainly, this mentality is proven effective in many pursuits. If you're going to run marathons or perform gymnastic

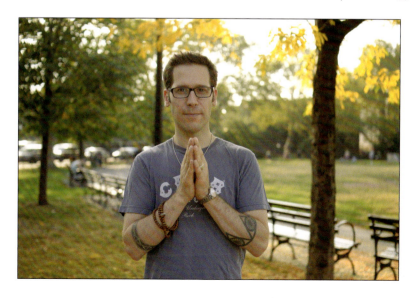

feats, then some amount of 'no pain, no gain' is likely going to be required to accomplish that task. But if what we are after is functional body health, then a see-how-far-we-can-push-the-limits mentality is counterproductive.

If we make yoga practice into hard work that never ends and never succumbs, rather than a forgiving effort that is easily and readily enjoyed, we paint our experience of life in the same unyielding hue.

The ultimate effect of both the *hard work* mindset and ever-challenging forms is the lasting impression of things never being enough and there always being more to do.

In both practice and life, the work does not need to be unnecessarily hard. Efforts in practice translate into our behaviors in myriad ways, and, more often than not, temperance is warranted.

Yes, I sometimes feel challenged by the life that is before me, sometimes I am overwhelmed. But being overly forceful with my body, or in life, has proven to be unhelpful in meeting the burdens that life bestows. I do not need to push my body hard in order to be well, and the efforts I make to meet the challenges that arise do not need to be a struggle."

J. Brown reminds me to ease up on my physical practice and myself. Even though you are likely wondering why I needed so many unique voices to shift my life, I'm wondering how I ever did it before I had them. Healthy life partners *were* what I was missing.

The problem is, once we're in a place where we're not seeing the truth, we don't want to experience the perceived pain required to challenge ourselves. It's not easy, but you can do it. *Accountability is a spiritual warrior's superpower.* Wouldn't you love to take your spiritual life to the next level of consciousness? The first step is to figure out who you are listening to. One teacher I listen to is Ashley Puran Aiken-Redon. She's become a trusted source of inspiration.

Ashley Puran Aiken-Redon

"Yoga has taught me *love*, it has taught me to know my Self, to accept it, to be at peace with it, and to own it unapologetically. It has taught me the true meaning of compassion and grace. It has taught me courage, discipline, and strength. It has taught me the infinite power of music, mantra, and sound. It has taught me awareness, presence, and acceptance. It has taught me to disidentify with my ego. It has taught me to be a better human being, to recognize my oneness with all, and so to see and love myself and all others, all else in this world, as *one*.

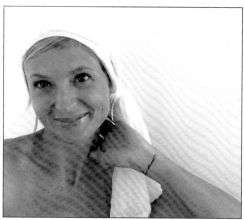

Yoga is for everyone. Yoga is your experience. It's about diving deeply within and truly making it your own personal experience. There are no expectations, no judgments, no limitations . . . it's about going to that place deep within your Being, where you find yourself at the very heart of the Universe, it's about going *home* to that place inside of you where stillness and peace reign and all is well. It's always been there, though we all too often forget, and it can never leave you, so dive deeply and remember this truth always!

Yoga keeps me balanced and in the flow of the present moment. It keeps me tuned in to my highest Self and teaches me to act from a place of heightened awareness and elevated consciousness."

Ashley's Kundalini practice comes from a place of love and authenticity. I know now that I was hiding my light, that I feared stepping into my divine greatness. Think about how it feels when you are in a safe space to just be yourself. I had lost that. I feared I would forever be stuck in the darkness of someone else's chaos. I had given up on myself. I was isolated, and alone.

What I needed was a loving environment and time to become aware and accountable. When I first heard Elena Brower speak about "articulating and loving the darkest aspects of ourselves," I was impressed with her raw vulnerability and eloquent insights. Elena taught me that accountability takes courage, but is incredibly loving and powerful.

Elena Brower

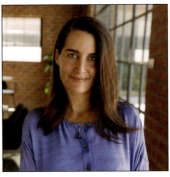

Pete Longworth

"Yoga has taught me to remain a student for the rest of my life. To continue asking for help, feedback, teachings, and guidance. It's also taught me to hear and trust my own intuition.

I use yoga to locate my breathing. It's the simplest and most rudimentary way to see my state—but it's also the key to the subtlest resonances in my being.

When I'm presented with a mental, emotional, or physical challenge, I am certain to open my mat during those times every morning. It helps me listen, love, stay open, and stay inquisitive. My practice is my beacon and my healing."

Change is hard, but I was stronger than I knew. So are you. Teachers like Elena helped launch me onto a quest to excavate my past and come to love myself, flaws and all. To have the courage to grow.

There's an incredible moment when you realize that growth might be easier than you think. Just reading and embodying the idea that yoga brings magic to your life, as Jacoby shared, encourages me to get to yoga daily. No excuses. You can carve out the time. Make yourself a priority. Schedule yoga on your calendar as a meeting if that makes you feel better. I've found that saying hello to other students motivates me to show up, because I look forward to seeing new friends. I also have taken the time to express my appreciation for the teachers and get to know them so that they are invested in my progress. Tell the teacher if you have any injuries and what you are hoping to accomplish in their class. You'll be amazed at how excited they are by your goals.

The teachers in this book are dedicated to your growth. They thrive when you do. They want you to love your experience on your journey. That is why they teach yoga. Yoga is the most powerful system I know to offer you a lifetime of less stress and a healthy direction for a balanced life. You are designing your life. Accepting accountability, your life begins to change. Your reality is created by the choices you are making.

I needed professional help in a safe, caring environment. If you need that, your yoga practice will only enhance that work. What are you waiting for? Reach down deep into your heart and ask yourself if you are worth it. You are. Walking away from what doesn't serve your soul is a behavior that can be learned. You don't have to struggle in isolation. When you find that things are becoming un-manageable, reach out to your yoga teacher for guidance.

TOP 10 REASONS TO GET TO KNOW YOUR YOGA TEACHER:

1. They help you sort out and clarify your values.

2. They help you achieve a better, richer life. Strength and flexibility are guaranteed, but it's the mental benefits that will keep you coming back for more.

3. Good teachers work hard to get you moving toward what you desire quickly.

4. They are experts at changing behavior.

5. Their value is measurable—you will see progress quickly. Great teachers point the way, allowing you to discover insights for yourself.

6. Even if you are comfortable, yoga and a "real deal" teacher can help you step out of your comfort zone. Here's the truth: there's only growth when you are out of your comfort zone. Great teachers make change attainable in a safe way.

7. A yoga teacher will hold space for you to name your fears, give you tools to act despite them, and change the way you feel about them.

8. A great teacher will show you how to listen to your intuition and apply that to your life.

9. Having someone validate your success and progress can be empowering. Your success will be acknowledged and celebrated.

10. Get yourself back on track. If you have been engaging in destructive behaviors, a teacher can guide you back to a healthy path. To have the courage to ask for help is a sign of someone who is ready to do the work. A teacher can listen to your issues in an unbiased and supportive manner and help you with an action plan.

Make sure and check their credentials. Do your homework. Ask the studio or gym if they are certified. Certifications matter. Even if it's yoga in the park that you found on a social site, they should be proud to share with you how long they have been teaching, where they studied, and by whom they are certified. In the new social online world, there are many peacocks posing in dangerous positions because they saw someone else do it. Proper alignment and attention could make all the difference in how long you practice. You don't want torn muscles, blown-out shoulders, or your knees replaced because of unhealthy sequencing. Learn from the best, and you'll practice for life. Once you've studied your road map, you're on your way to living a life full of potential.

CHAPTER 4

Staying Real

To say that my next treatment center was an abject nightmare would be sugarcoating it. Inasmuch as TC1 provided a loving and safe environment where I'd felt supported and understood *for the first time*, TC2 could not have felt less safe. Here, when I used my recently discovered voice to speak up for myself, I found myself stripped of all privileges. Worse, they summoned my husband, telling him I had been "causing trouble."

TREATMENT CENTER TWO (TC2)

Everything became clear when my husband showed up. I recall it vividly. I waited in the front room, holding a drawing I'd made in art therapy. "I'm so glad to see you," I proclaimed in an upbeat manner when he walked in. "I'm not glad to see you," he deadpanned.

I knew then, unequivocally, that my best friend of twenty-five years had never been my friend at all.

He'd brought along the Pittsburgh therapist. This same woman who'd once escorted my husband out of the room for yelling at me now appeared to be yet another person on his payroll. Oh, it's hard to be married to a successful man, all right! *My abusers were back. Horrified and retraumatized, I froze.*

FAMILY WEEK

One bright spot brewed on the horizon: family week. I longed to see my daughters. The mere thought of it fueled me to no end; I'm not shy to tell you, I cried tears of joy when I found out they were coming.

However, following my husband's disastrous visit, they cancelled my family week. *I cried and pleaded and begged to be allowed see my daughters. Denied.*

I knew at that moment that I was under the complete control of my husband and that his money and power had erased me.

Distraught beyond words, I shared what happened with another patient, who attempted to comfort me. For this violation of a new "rule"—a rule that had been handed down after my husband's visit (which was disturbing considering I had just reclaimed my right to speak up)—that I not be allowed to speak to anyone, I was asked to leave the center. My distress now at a peak, I called, *of all people*, my husband. To my shock and bewilderment, he told me, "If you don't get back in, we're divorced."

Considering for a moment that *I was the one who'd said I wanted a divorce*, I sheepishly went back to the center and begged to be readmitted. Make no mistake, I wanted out. But I wanted my daughters more. And I believed this was the only way to get back to them.

They refused. My husband changed the locks on our home in Pittsburgh—I've never been allowed back since that day. The only corner on the planet I could call my own was a condo in Arizona I'd purchased years earlier. So I headed there.

SPIRITUAL WARRIOR WISDOM

The abusers tried to eliminate my voice, once again, and I feared that I would remain under someone else's control unless I took the wheel of my own life. I know now that fear of the unknown is a wasted emotion that keeps you feeling sabotaged. This is what Valerie Goodman had to learn. Stepping back and *seeing the bigger picture* allowed her to move forward.

Valerie Goodman

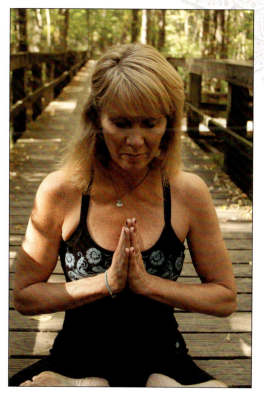

"Know you have a purpose. The physical practice is a cobble-stoned pathway into the unexpected. You may teeter on the rocks initially, but, somewhere along the way, you learn how to walk.

Yoga is a way of seeing the Light ease through your *cracks*—physical, mental, emotional—and you build the strength you need.

Yoga keeps me stable, balanced, inspired to do more, to be more. It has made me strong in both tangible and intangible ways. Yoga has a delicious way of distracting my mind long enough for the reminder of what I need to do. It makes it possible for me to detach, step back, and see the bigger picture.

Life before brain surgery at forty, I dreamed while sleeping. After being pushed to the edge, my Higher Power illuminated the road I needed to take. I would not change one previous moment, because I know each was necessary to be here now. And ever since that one discovery of yoga . . . my dreams are experienced while awake. Pretty sweet."

Yoga *opened a mental door* that Valerie didn't know existed. She became more self-aware. One of the best things about owning your life is that self-awareness allows you to acknowledge your situation and make changes. I didn't need another crash. I needed to use yoga to empower myself. To understand and embrace my reality, just like Karina Ayn Mirsky did when facing her profound challenge.

STAYING REAL

Karina Ayn Mirsky

"Yoga saved my life. One of the most profound challenges I've faced was being diagnosed with lymphatic cancer when I was twenty-seven years old.

When I was twenty-six, I started having panic attacks. So, I went to see a psychotherapist, who said that sometimes anxiety is something in us that 'wants to be known.' So I meditated on the anxiety and asked it to reveal to me what it wanted me to know. The anxiety started to hone in on my left tonsil, which had been chronically inflamed for years but was now larger than it ever had been. So I went to the doctor. I was sent home with some antibiotics. I went back a second time a few weeks later and was sent home with some anti-inflammatory medication.

When the anxiety continued to increase, I meditated on the tonsil, asking it what it wanted. It was made clear to me in meditation that my tonsils needed to come out. On my third visit to the doctor, I begged to be referred to a specialist. He removed the tonsils. The tonsillectomy revealed that the left tonsil contained a malignant lymphoma.

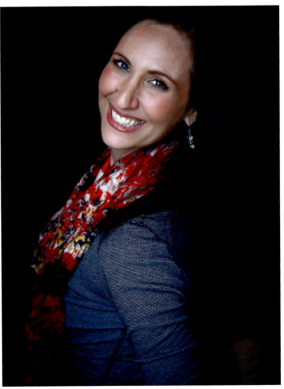

Yogic practices like yoga Nidra and mantra meditation were my lifeline as I endured six months of invasive chemotherapy. Today, I have a clean bill of health and coach others facing similar life challenges.

There are as many perceptions of reality as there are people. Yoga taught me the value in observing my thoughts and challenging my beliefs. Self-inquiry has given me greater understanding, acceptance, and compassion for myself and others. It has empowered me with a capacity to transform limiting thoughts and choose how I want to experience the world. Yoga has also taught me that there is a difference between pain and suffering. I've learned that pain regulation starts with present moment awareness and acceptance and compassion for what is. I've learned that both the mind and the body can be harmonized through harmonizing the patterns of breath. I've also realized that there is a Self within me that is always clear, calm, and tranquil. So yoga has given me the tools to self-regulate and imbued me with a sense of trust that I always am and will always be okay.

Yoga isn't what most people think it is. It's not limited to the physical practices. Yoga is about learning how to embody true happiness and contentment. It can support anyone, even those who aren't able to do, or interested in doing, yoga postures. Yoga is a methodology to reduce suffering and empower individuals with self-understanding and choice. It is a way to elevate one's consciousness above fear and pain. *You don't ever have to do a yoga pose to practice yoga.* All you need is a sincere desire to be happy and a willingness to change your life for the better."

Karina teaches that you have the power to choose who you want to be and how you want to feel and act in any given moment. Your reality is created by you from the choices you make. Although I claimed that power at TC1, I still had a lot to learn about knowing who I was. It was time. Just like Robin Afinowich learned that yoga teaches us about all aspects of ourselves, our lives, and the choices we make to create those.

Robin Afinowich

"Everything in yoga is a metaphor for life. Yoga has something to teach us every single time we step onto the mat or sit in meditation. Yoga teaches us to be present in, accepting of, and compassionate to whatever surfaces. It teaches us to be attuned to the dynamic interplay of mind, body, energy, and spirit, and to find awe in and reverence for the delicate dance of self-embodiment that creates our livelihood.

Yoga teaches us about unconditional love, that we are good enough even when it's hard to breathe, focus, or stand on one leg. Yoga teaches us to come to the edge of discomfort and meet it with tenderness, grace, and gratitude, for without the rough edges, our soul couldn't polish. It is medicine and science, psyche and spirit, energetic alchemy, and a magical mystery all in one. Yoga teaches us that the power isn't in the posture, but rather in the integrity and intention beneath the muscle and bone. Power is standing at the center of ourselves and knowing, without shame or fear, who we are.

Yoga helps us be better mothers, wives, friends, healers, and more conscious beings in the world. Yoga reminds us about impermanence; we build a posture and deconstruct a posture only to build another. It reminds us that everything is changing and evolving, and yet in the space between thoughts and motion, there are landscapes of stillness that invite us in to rest, to witness, to be. *Yoga teaches us to be delicately aware of our sacred life.*

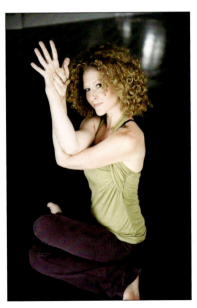

When experiencing challenge, turn to deep yoga. It centers you, relaxes you, and provides a space for the sacred pause, that zone where you can slip into the art of mindfulness and be more aware of your responses and reactions. Other times, you come to the mat to sweat out the challenges, to check out of your mind completely, and drop into precision of form and function, energy, and flow.

Meditation helps you connect to something bigger than your thoughts or challenges, something more universal and innately soothing.

When I was diagnosed with cancer, I sat and had tea with my fears, I talked to them, accepted them, moved through them. The practice taught me to listen, trust, pay attention, and embrace the journey, no matter how difficult.

Yoga helps us overcome challenges by creating meaning and purpose in all that occurs, the good and the bad. The greatest teacher is the biggest challenge; I often consider cancer a guru. *Yoga has allowed me to listen to the whispers of wisdom that hide in the shadows.* In these seemingly ominous and dark pockets of life, there breathes black-cloaked teachers patiently waiting to share their messages with us, and when we approach them with faith, humility, and reverence, they remove their hoods and look at us tenderly through the same eyes of God that dwell in the lighter days of my life. When we give our challenges or suffering meaning, they become our allies for awakening.

Yoga is for those who are looking for self-acceptance, inner peace, spiritual connection, and healing of body and mind. All of us."

Robin Afinowich is an advocate of getting real with yourself. Get specific about what choices you make in this world, because those choices carry responsibilities. When you consistently choose the right thoughts and behavior—with discipline—a healthy path emerges. Robin Martin learned with discipline how to manage her breathing, something she uses to manage her fears and anxieties.

Robin Martin

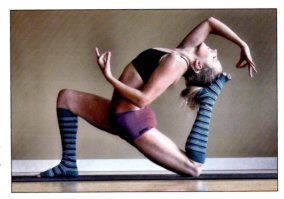

"I battled anxiety in college and had a fear of flying for many years. I've never taken anxiety medication, but there was a time where I probably could have used it. I learned to control my anxiety with my breath. It's a gift that has changed my life. I take time on my mat to find my breath and let go of the thoughts or ideas that challenge me.

My fear of flying kept me grounded, mostly fearing I would have a panic attack midflight. I now travel comfortably, knowing I'm in control of my breath: therefore, I'm in control of anxiety.

The moment I knew I wanted to be a teacher was when I finally realized how yoga affected me beyond the studio. It was something I wanted to share with others so that they might have the same experience: the ability to find a moving meditation, and to leave class with a sense of lightness of being.

Yoga has taught me that I can control my anxiety. Yoga also taught me that I can let go of the things that don't serve me, and I can be a wife and mother, but be myself first. Yoga has opened my mind and eyes to the world around me. I want to see and experience as much as possible, give back as much as I can.

Yoga settles my mind. If I have a challenging situation in my life, I take time on my mat to find my breath and let go of the thoughts or ideas that challenge me. I can think more clearly following a yoga practice. I won't react with emotion or frustration, but rather with a sense of calm. Challenges seem less challenging after a yoga practice.

Yoga is about the mind first, the physical body second. Quieting the mind is a gift. Find time to quiet the mind each day, and you will be a gift to others around you."

Robin's advice about "letting go of the things that don't serve you" tells me that we can be limitless. The clarity and simplicity of the message Robin shares is invaluable.

Karolina Krawczyk-Sharma has a similar message about the need to get specific about your wants and needs in life. That it's perfectly normal to stop and question where you're at in your life design.

Karolina Krawczyk-Sharma

"I am a diabetic, Type 1. I got diagnosed at the age of fifteen. Looking for support for my body, and believing that there is some healing potential somewhere in the world, I discovered yoga. I was disappointed with conventional medicine. I was scared, depressed, and felt guilty. Yoga brought a new perspective to my disease. I discovered that I can feel healthy, energetic, happy. . . . The healing power of yoga is not on the surface, but it is on the deepest level.

First of all, yoga taught me that we are perfect the way we are, and that life is good. Not always easy, not always according to our preconceptions of it, but always good.

It shows and reminds us that the Universe is providing us with everything we need, and everyone we can learn from. Yoga also taught me that love is the answer.

It brought me home. It brought me back to my body, to its health. It brought me to my inner belief that it is okay to be me. It reminded me that I have the right to be happy, live my life, and follow my dreams.

Yoga teaches reflection. Whenever I face any challenge, I ask myself: What can I learn from it? How can I make the situation better, or at least beneficial? Or what can I do to handle it the best I can? If we cannot change the situation, at least we can change our perspective on it. We need to trust that there are some reasons why certain things happen to us, and that they are exactly what we need. We might not see it at once, but after a while we can find positive sides of everything.

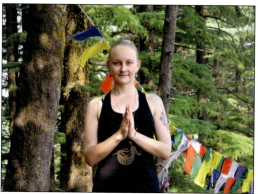

See, that's the case of my *disease*—you can make drama out of it, but to be honest, it brought me to where I stand today: happy, healthy, smiling, and enjoying my life. Before I became diabetic, my diet was horribly unconscious, my life was a mess, my relations full of tension, my every day full of worries. But this experience allowed me to discover a new perspective, take care of myself, being more aware, more careful how I distribute my energy in life, how I spend my limited time, who is around me. . . . My choices today make me feel much better and happier."

Karolina learned, though yoga, how to step back and look at her life from a healthy perspective. The sense of betrayal I felt at TC2 felt like a scab had been ripped off a wound that was just starting to heal. Life, even with a regular yoga practice, will continue to give you challenges. I may have had new tools, but I was not yet skillful in applying them. Deborah Burkman espouses the same philosophical belief that I do—that suffering is inherent in the human experience. With yoga, though, you can learn new, skillful ways of living to your highest potential, despite what challenges come your way.

Deborah Burkman

"I was diagnosed with breast cancer ten days before my wedding.

One of the most difficult things had to do with waiting one month to find out how life-threatening my cancer was. At first, I had a 'poor me' moment. 'Why now?' Those thoughts faded, and then I found it difficult to stop my mind from obsessing on the 'what-ifs.' Then I had a momentous shift. I was driving in my car and thought about the survivors of the Boston marathon bombing, many of whom were athletes who lost limbs. I realized they had a choice. They could spend the rest of their lives living as a victim and holding on to anger for all that was taken from them. Or, they could see the miracle of their survival and accept their new life and do something with it.

Although I realized that my situation was not as severe, I too had that same choice. My daily asana practice helped me to see when my mind went into imagination and 'what-ifs.' My breath helped bring me back to the present moment and what I knew and didn't know. The weekend of my wedding was perfect. I had the awareness that nothing is guaranteed, and each moment with my husband and family and friends was precious. It doesn't mean the fear went away, but there was room for both the beauty in the present moment and my fear.

There is suffering in life. The best tool humans have to deal with this suffering is yoga. When you have a stable body and mind and a strong sense of self, when hardships come, you are more skillful with them. You will move through hardship instead of being stuck in it. Your sense of self is larger than any one problem that comes your way. Yoga does not prevent pain, it helps you manage it. Your pain is not unique. Instead of asking, 'Why me?' the true question is 'Why not me?'

Focus on your breath. The breath serves as an anchor to a turbulent mind. Coming back to the breath allows you to see where your mind is taking you.

You will begin to understand yourself better once you can see which thought patterns emerge. Mood is affected by circumstance, and self-perception can be influenced by others.

Yoga teaches the value of *Kaivalyam*, which is Sanskrit for independence from one's own thoughts, feelings, circumstance, and other people. For example, instead of giving in to doubt and fear while in a challenging yoga posture, learn to access faith and courage instead. This independence from thoughts leads to a stronger sense of self. These benefits began to surface only after I developed a daily practice. The results of a daily discipline are cumulative, and only over time are the results profound. The discipline developed in this area begins to manifest in other areas, as well. However, the benefits of this independence are not a constant. There can be moments of focus and clarity, but still times of confusion and doubt. Yoga teaches compassion when there are unskillful actions. Notice, and get back on track.

Study the *Yogasūtra*. If things don't go your way, remember *Isvara Pranidhanai* and surrender to the larger reality. Work with the things you can control and accept the things you can't. Yoga helps to discern the difference.

Yoga helps let go of tightness and restriction around challenge. When you are relaxed, you can see more clearly what is actually happening. Trust that you can move through the hard times. Accept that you live in an imperfect world and stay connected to what is meaningful in the larger picture of life."

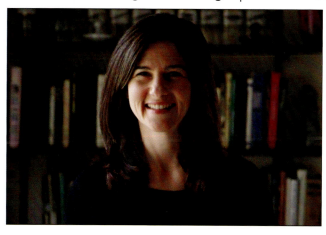

Deborah reminds me that life is ever-changing and change is hard. But if we embrace the idea that although there is struggle in change, there is also beauty and opportunity, then we experience a chance for a real-life shift.

At TC1, I was given an opportunity to change, to become authentic, conscious. But I needed to turn that opportunity into reality. Mas Vidal taught me to dig deep into my practice and to find ways to understand how to make it a daily exploration into living from a place that was real, that was authentic. *To be free.*

Mas Vidal

"A number of events kept expanding my heart. The first one was in college in Florida, when my heart was broken open by a college girlfriend. I realized at that point that love and happiness could not be dependent on a person or thing. I wanted to know a love that was beyond shape and form, name, or brand. Hence my search began, but many old habits remained, and I ended up in jail on New Year's night, which ended up with a load of community service hours and some routine meetings with a counselor. I found out I could do those community service hours at Nonprofit Religious or Education organizations, and I chose SRF, or Self Realization Fellowship, the organization founded by the famous Hindu-Yogi Guru Paramahansa Yogananda, author of *Autobiography of a Yogi*. Not only did I enjoy serving there, in the gardens landscaping, cooking, and doing whatever the monks asked me to do, but I quickly accomplished the community service hours and decided to keep serving there, to study the teachings and learn about yoga and about meditation.

Physically, use asana yoga to improve circulation, remove muscular tension, and improve flexibility. For mental and emotional challenges, practice kriya yoga meditation and offer prayers to Lakshmi Devi and to Shiva in the form of Nataraj. Pray deeply for understanding of your karma through the experiences you are confronted with each day in the world. My practice of yoga is alive in that I try to see the Divine hand behind the things I don't understand. Yoga is about uniting with God through nature. For me, God and nature are not separate. Nature and our subtle intuitive feelings are God's language that provides consolation and guidance back to our true source.

Observe the three Cs of a yoga lifestyle. First is 'commitment,' and once we make a commitment to practice yoga, we must stick to it for our entire life. It's not a part-time thing, it's all the time. It's at home, at work, in society, personally, and in our heads. We must remain committed to the idea that we are not the body, nor the mind, we are a soul, a Divine being filled with light, love, and peace. That's commitment! Second is 'concentration.' We must have the power of attention, focus, and presence of mind in anything we do. No multitasking will work. Concentration is the key to success in any field, and especially in the mind-body medicine and Ayurveda. When the winds of thoughts blow through the mind, it can be disastrous, but when the mental thoughts are calmed and focused, then we have mastery over the I/me/mine illusions, and we are free. The last one is 'consistency' in anything we do, and especially in yoga sadhana. It's not how much we do something, but how consistently we do it. What we do consistently the most, we ultimately become that.

Try yoga in any way that you can or that appeals to you. When the student is ready, the teacher will appear. Try yoga in the most convenient way possible; find it near your home, online, in books, and wherever you are ready and willing to embrace it. Yoga has many sides and can begin with meditation, mantra, breathing, or even serving others through some community work. Or even easier, just repeat the words: 'I am love, I am light, I am peace.' That's also yoga, as we affirm our true essence. *Practice yoga, live Ayurveda, and let the Divine take care of the rest."*

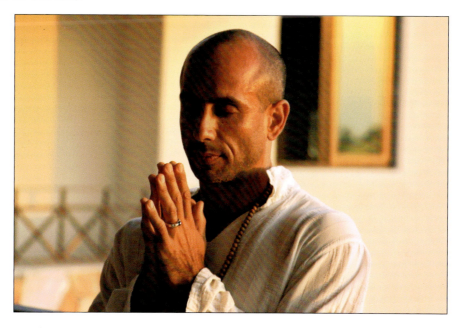

Mas instructs that yoga is a way of being. Cultivating body, mind, and spirit are worthwhile because you're valuable. Valuable indeed. Somewhere along the way, I had forgotten I was a valuable person, but no more. If we combine choice with what Mas tells us, we should choose to surround ourselves with people who see the real us, the beautiful us.

THE YOGINI IN ME NEEDS TO SHARE . . .

Elizabeth Gilbert, Author of *Eat Pray Love*, encouraged me to write this book. I met Gilbert in Arizona, shortly after arriving. I was no way near ready to step into the wisdom that was unfolding before me moment to moment once I had solitude. I found her encouragement enlightening because she openly shared that her other books up until that point had gone unnoticed.

When I met her, I hadn't even dreamed of my Yoga Road Trip. I had not totally reclaimed my voice and power yet. But I got on the on-ramp of my new journey. Staying real. Embracing vulnerability, I was courageously excavating my truth. Looking hard at where I was in my life, I knew speaking up for women who felt voiceless would help me heal. I didn't know how yet. I had to look inside more and search for the answer. When was the last time you took a long, hard look at where you are at and where you are going?

Along with the other voices I have gathered for you, I have shared my experience in the hope that you remember that the choices you make in this world impact not only yourself, but also those around you. Once you have started practicing yoga postures, you learn that the goal of the physical practice is to get to the meditative part: Savasana, or Corpse Pose.

If you want to radically change your life, you will become aware of the voice of your internal self during Savasana. Sometimes, this is the most challenging pose. By being inquisitive about what happens while you are still and quiet, you will take all of the wisdom of the practice with you into your day.

It's important to remember that this is a practice. It's also not intended to be a one-off or easy. It's effective, though, for bringing the peace and balance that you seek.

Once you become still, all types of *stuff* surfaces. It isn't always pretty, that's for sure. But by acknowledging the situation you are in and looking at the behaviors that result from that, you have the option to change the things that no longer serve you.

Hate speech is not free speech. Smile in the understanding that freedom from the internal critic is possible. If you're feeling like the chitchat that is going on in your mind isn't your best friend, then notice how much of your day you stay in that. Even dropping some of the negativity and hopefully replacing it with positive statements will bring more joy. Your relationships will improve. Your mood will change. Everything from productivity to connectivity will change.

Once you make this a practice, you start to notice it more. How do you speak to yourself? With loving kindness, or criticism? *Those who control their thoughts control their lives.* Meditation and yoga go hand in hand because you will learn to tune in to that inner voice and even talk back to it.

Think of it as a loving partner. Your body is a great source of wisdom and creativity. For instance, think about how long it took you to learn to walk. Babies try over and over to get upright and moving, never giving up. When you are consistently showing up on your mat, never giving up, your loving partner will support you.

Your thoughts, your intellectual self, behave the way you choose. Once you've gotten clear about the behaviors you wish to embody, your intellect becomes a part of the trip. If you ignore the behaviors that result from your inability to design your day, you might end up crashing, like I did. For me, one of the skills I wish I'd acquired sooner is listening to that voice.

A loving partner—and I mean yourself as your loving partner—is the key. Make a conscious choice to get quiet. To listen. Be open to examining how this stillness can bring awareness to your day. Figure out your most effective way to do that. Expend the time and energy to lean into the stillness. Bring your best self to the moment by tuning in to your inner voice. Listen. Breathe. When you are in a state of connectivity, trust what you hear. Act on that information. Try again and again.

HERE ARE SOME THINGS YOU CAN DO RIGHT NOW TO ENHANCE YOUR AWARENESS:

1. Dedicate a small place in your home to be still. Clear everything out of your view except for either a candle or a journal. Start with five minutes. You might try and focus on the candle, or simply close your eyes. Perhaps say to yourself, "Breathing in, breathing out," and see if you can stay with that. Set a timer if you need to. Breathe. Listen.

2. If sitting still is challenging, consider staying in Savasana at the end of practice for longer than five minutes. Many studios now rush people out of class, when traditionally Savasana used to be a least twenty minutes. Make a conscious choice when you can to stay with the intent of examining your internal voice. The key is not to judge the thoughts. Simply witness. Use a voice app to quickly jot down your thoughts if you're rushing off to the rest of your day.

3. Figure out how you want to record the thoughts to refer to. Journaling, even a line or two, brings huge results. At the end of the day, reflect on what you wrote. If you forget, pick up your journal and read it on the weekend or when you have quiet time to reflect. See if what you are thinking is enhancing or detracting from your day.

4. When you consistently connect your experience, thoughts, and feelings while practicing yoga with your behaviors off the mat, you can tune in to being accountable for your life. If you're the kind of person who believes that you already have all the answers, this could be quite the challenge. Be open to the idea that you might learn something new. We're human. You're either standing still or growing. Change is a given. What's it going to be? This isn't to torture you. It doesn't have to be a big pill to swallow; it might be the best thing you've ever done for yourself. Wrong or right is judgment, I encourage you to look at it as an assessment. Listening to, and getting to be best friends with, your inner voice will bring great rewards. You deserve a healthy life. Tune in. Wake up. Soulful goals take practice.

CHAPTER 5

Embracing the Potholes and Detours of Life

I can't say I remember much about the drive from New Mexico to Arizona. Still numb, I do remember rolling down the windows near Show Low, Arizona.

ARIZONA-BOUND

New Mexico and Arizona are mostly brown and dry in July, but at that elevation, the trees looked so green.

I turned the key in the door of my condo in Scottsdale on July 5th. For the first time since that fateful day in St. Barts, I felt euphoric. Finally, I had my freedom.

A LOFTY PLAN IS HATCHED

To bolster self-worth, I created a simple routine that was built around one thing: my daily yoga practice. I don't remember who said, "When the student is ready, the teacher appears," but it has rung true for me since I started practicing yoga some thirty-seven-plus years ago. No matter where I live or what language is spoken, no matter if it's outside or inside, big or small studio, mat-to-mat or a handful of people, the right teacher always seems to appear. *Wherever I lay my mat, that's my home.*

However, much work lay ahead. While at TC1, I'd had an epiphany: I decided to be the one to break the cycle of abuse that had plagued generations of my family. I committed to myself to be the antitrauma and antiabuse superhero! *A lofty goal, for sure. So, it's no surprise I took up flying.*

FLYING HIGH

One day, while driving home from yoga, I stalled my car. It was my elder daughter's birthday, and I missed her horribly. I'd been hopeful she'd acknowledge the present I'd sent, but I hadn't heard from her. I feared a whole new dynamic was surfacing as my gifts, emails, voicemails, and letters were all going unanswered.

The top down in my convertible, I pulled up at a red light and looked up at the sky. With tears streaming down my face, I yelled, "God, please give me a sign that everything's going to be okay!"

Mortified, I realized that the people in the car next to me were staring. Embarrassed to be seen with my *mask* off, I jammed the car into gear . . . and stalled it. Now totally humiliated, I cranked it up again, sped onto a street I didn't know, and came to a dead end at a small, private airport.

Struck by inspiration, I got out and walked inside the office to inquire about flying lessons. I took my first lesson that day.

Flying became a great adventure for me. Wonderful and exhilarating and liberating. Turns out, I excelled at it.

A few weeks later, our attorney arrived on my husband's jet, handed me a stack of divorce papers, and, with the stroke of a pen, a chapter of my life closed.

In a brief phone conversation, my now ex-husband insisted we be "just like Bruce and Demi." At the time, Bruce Willis and Demi Moore were all over the media looking like the happiest and best of friends throughout their divorce. My ex-husband wanted our divorce to look like an equally amicable parting, because public appearances meant everything to him.

Still raw, being friends was the last thing on my mind. My only focus: my new life and salvaging the only thing about my old one that mattered—my relationship with my daughters. But I believed that being friendly with my ex-husband would help me reconnect with them. *Wrong, once again.*

SPIRITUAL WARRIOR WISDOM

Pain has been a great teacher in my life. I originally began my yoga practice because I suffered from chronic back pain. Are you expecting someone else to make your pain go away, or are you exhausting every option you can find to live in optimal health? Spoiler alert: potholes and detours on your road to wellness should be expected.

As with learning any new skill, it takes practice. Be gentle with yourself. Be encouraging to yourself. Be firm, yet determined. When you view the world filtered through past events, you allow your past to control and dictate both your present and your future. I had as much unlearning as learning to do. Ally Hamilton reminds me that we're organic, ever-changing, and growing when we use yoga as a healthy partner.

Ally Hamilton

"Yoga has taught me that we are always in process. We're never *done* until that final exhale. Yoga is a philosophy, an art, and a science of traveling inward. We quiet the storm that's raging in the mind. We get it to settle into the present instead of forever heading into the past and future. We create some space between our thoughts, and in that space, we usually discover our own intuition, and a lot of peace. Yoga gives us the tools to face reality as it is, and to face ourselves as we are. And to get to work healing if we're in need of that. Further, it gives us the power to let go of the ideas and tendencies that aren't serving us. It strips away anything that is inauthentic, whether it's a job we have, relationships we're in, coping mechanisms that are weakening us, or stories we're telling ourselves about why we are the way we are, which may be old, ingrained, and untrue.

Personally, yoga has taught me to seek out and work with the truth, and when I say, 'the truth,' I don't mean there's one truth for all of us; I mean, what is true for me. What is true for the people closest to me. I used to chase happiness, long for it, strive away, and come up empty, defeated, and disappointed in others or myself. It took years, but yoga has given me a hunger for what is real. Reality might break your heart sometimes; in fact, it probably will. But I'd rather be heartbroken than numb, or deluded.

Initially I thought I was finding a physical practice, but what I found was the foundation for living my life in a way that feels good.

Just know that we all have stuff. We all have history and issues, and ways we sabotage ourselves. True happiness is not an avoidance of pain; it's an ability to open to things as they are. You can't run from your pain, or deny it, or push it down; if you do, it owns you, you're a slave to it. Yoga gives us the tools to be brave and vulnerable at the same time. You can't change the world around you. You can't change what other people will do or want or say or need, but you can create a peaceful world within you. A compassionate, kind, aware, awake, honest world. Yoga gives us the tools to do that, and the beauty lies in this one fact: what you have within you is

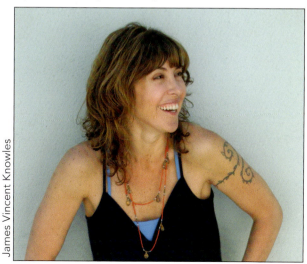

James Vincent Knowles

what you'll spread as you move through the world. So even though yoga is a gift you give to yourself, it's also a gift you bring to everyone you encounter. We change the world around us by changing the world within us.

Nonreactivity is one of the main things we work on in yoga. The ability to lean into intense sensation, and keep breathing, and stay curious about our experience. It might not seem obvious, but the burning sensation in your quadriceps from holding a lunge for ten deep breaths will serve you the next time you feel enraged, jealous, lonely, fearful, or anxious. When we talk about these difficult emotions, what we're really referring to is the sensations they create in our bodies. The pain and ache that settle over the heart and reside in the chest when we feel rejected or discarded. The racing heart, shallow breath, clenched jaw, and tight shoulders we experience when we're angry. The sick feeling in the pit of our stomach when we feel jealous. Training your mind and your nervous system to breathe through intense sensation on your mat will absolutely translate to challenging moments in your life. There's no separation, it's the same stuff."

The wisdom of bringing the physical back to the emotional is a unique perspective that Ally taught me. Your emotions aren't stupid. Joy, sadness, anger—all emotions are important. Connecting body and emotions is a "deep journey" inward, as Liz Terry shares.

Liz Terry

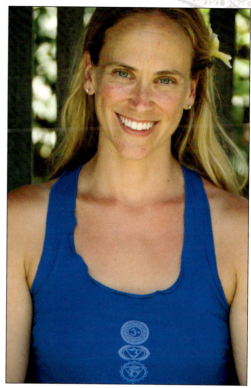

"My process began in the midst of despair. At twenty-four, I was anxious, a perfectionist, a control freak, and completely exhausted. I know I was led to yoga through divine intervention because I simply stumbled upon it one day without really knowing what it was.

I've learned to let things be. Instead of believing that I have control over what life will throw at me, I now understand that the only thing I can control is the way I react to what life throws at me. Yoga has taken me on a journey deep within myself, so that I have begun to appreciate what life should offer in each moment. When I get pulled away from myself, I head back to my mat for reflection, introspection, and love toward myself and those whom I've been fortunate enough to meet along my path.

Most people start their yogic journey through asana, or the physical aspect of yoga, and the body can teach us so much about ourselves. It may be scary at first, but once you get on board, once you start to notice and observe all the ups and downs, the experience is necessary and worth the ride. Once we begin to allow ourselves to connect to the body through asana, there's just no turning back.

The simple act of stillness has created a shift so deep within my mind and body, I can't help but feel more connected to my source."

Letting go, letting things be—loosening your perception of what you need to control: all wise counsel from a loving friend. No longer willing to check out of my days, I was letting go of old patterns and behaviors. Life is meant to be lived, open, and fearless, as Lori Tindall came to understand and embrace.

Lori Tindall

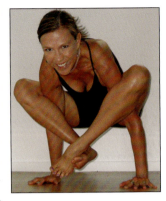

"I kept my metaphysical life a secret growing up, and switching gears to open up with it, even to this day, has been challenging. I've felt conflicted between the 'woo-woo' aspects of my metaphysical life and my desire to be scientific and grounded in reality. I had felt my sporting and scientific life was separate from my yogic metaphysical life, and this separation left me feeling separated! It is perhaps this conflict within me that allows me to sort through the yoga practices in a more helpful manner now, but it wasn't until I was sitting at the Olympic Training Center in Colorado Springs 2000, listening to a presentation by a sports psychologist, that my conflicting worlds collided. As the psychologist was explaining the inner mental and emotional methods for triathlon, all I could hear was him describing Patanjali's yoga sutras. It was then that I started realizing my worlds were not separate from each other, but that it was society that might not have the understanding—yet. Now I have a fuller perspective on what being grounded in reality really means to me.

I was born with an inborn error in my immune system. This leaves me open to very serious, and sometimes life-threatening, infections. It's called Common Variable Immunodeficiency, but it's certainly not common. Yoga offers very resourceful tools to help with the difficulties in life. Yoga is about being calm and centered within the chaos of life.

The simplest technique of observing my breath and all that may arise is what I always come back to. I apply it to a difficult workout, while receiving a painful medical treatment, through illness, while driving and being frustrated with traffic, or within a pause during a difficult communication scenario. It's powerful in its simplicity but can be effective when applied with mental fortitude.

Life is a crazy roller coaster, and it can be both difficult and fun. If we deny this, then we deny life itself. Each time we go up on a scary section and we become more familiar with it, it becomes less scary, and it's from this experience that a calm center can arise. Yet it is through the scariness of the experience that we can be both exhilarated and changed. There is a duality in the experiences that gives us contrast and more definition. Once we rest in this greater understanding, we take our experiences for what they are: experiences! It's who we are and who we are becoming within the vastness of the Universe and our experiences; that is yoga."

Lori used yoga and observing her breath to embrace the ride of her life. Riding in the passenger seat no more, I may have felt raw at times, but I was all in now. There was no turning back. Yoga plays a pivotal part in allowing you to live at your peak potential, because you no longer get stuck in the potholes; you navigate around them. Meg Pearson figured out a new course for her life, just as you can.

Meg Pearson

"Having suffered with an eating disorder for over half my life, my journey of self-discovery began early. But my desire for change truly came to a head in the fall of 2010. It was then that I was going through the lowest point of my life, and after hitting the proverbial rock bottom, I knew that I had only one option; I chose to fight for my life.

I was bankrupt, unemployed, and depressed. My father was ill with fronto-temporal dementia and ALS, and the diseases' progressions were rapid. My

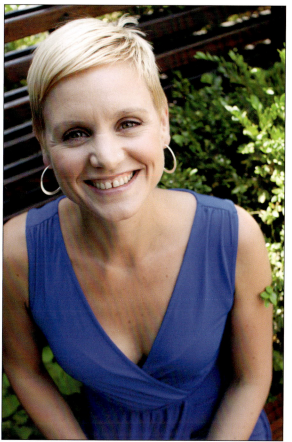

then (now ex-) fiancé and I had called off our wedding less than four months before the big day, and my heart ached in a way I had never known prior to then. Still ahead were my young nephew's brain tumor and surgery, and then the eventual passing of my dad at age sixty-three. But I persevered.

It was a rough go, but I made it through and lived to tell the tale. It *is* possible to move on from what may seem like the end of the line, it *is* okay to succumb to the pain, ask for help, and just be with yourself until you are prepared to move forward. Out of all my suffering, I could redirect my life and figure out a new course.

When I am having a stressful day, I take a PM practice break, and that always refocuses me.

However, I need not actually hit the mat in a physical sense to reap the benefits. Sometimes, I just breathe. Deep. And feel grateful. And that is all I need to ride things out. Acceptance is what is helpful. Choosing ahimsa, or acting in a nonharming way, helps to avoid unnecessary confrontation. *Yoga welcomes peace. And peace obliterates many of life's challenges.*

Yoga is not just a practice of moving through the asanas. It's a mental state. A thought process, and once you adopt it, life changes.

To someone who struggled with anorexia, bulimia, and functional alcoholism for close to eighteen years, yoga was a life changer. I learned that presence is perfection and imperfection. Just being, in the moment, in the body, in the world, is all you need. I can headstand or backbend my way out of any bad mood. As a matter of fact, I rarely get into those bad moods of the past anymore, so long as I am regularly practicing. Ten minutes, ninety minutes, it doesn't even matter. Show up, be who you are, where you are, and everything will fall into proper place. Be patient. With yourself, with others, with change. I have also discovered that I am awesome. So are you. We really rock.

There is a recipe for body love. I am a wellness warrior. Proud and free. Yoga is the key. To comfort. Physically and mentally and in your heart. Feel young and be young. Yoga will help you discover things about yourself you never knew possible. To appreciate things. To breathe more. To value more. To be more. To feel more.

I love knowing that I always have yoga in my toolbox. It is always a weapon of love tucked into my back pocket."

Peace is possible, as Meg discovered. Make peace with your past. Design your future. Monette Chilson believes there is much to learn, especially when it comes to messages we have gathered from the society we live in.

Monette Chilson

"I am a yoga teacher who chooses to focus my teaching on all eight limbs of yoga—the ethical practices, avoidances, postures, breath, withdrawal of senses, concentration, meditation, and union with the divine. *Sometimes our inner self is so much wiser than we realize.*

Yoga has taught me so many lessons, including humility, patience, gratitude, balance, and acceptance.

My yoga has taught me that all the notions of separation that we impose on our lives are false. There is no one part of my life that's spiritual. It's all spiritual. I learned to embody stillness, and at last I could relax and relish my newfound status as a human being, rather than a human doing!

You don't have to be flexible to do yoga. You don't have to be the yoga type. You don't have to wear Birkenstocks or become a vegetarian. You just show up, unroll your mat, and be present.

The media—even those outlets with the best intentions—make us think it's all about the yoga pants, the willowy body, and the way yoga makes us look. That's a lie. It's about how the body feels. You will learn a whole new definition of sexy, one not based on external looks or validation, but one born of a humming that starts from deep within, making you feel alive and vital. Cultivating this energy and carrying it with you into the world is a thousand times more important than striking a pose that looks like the one on that glossy magazine cover.

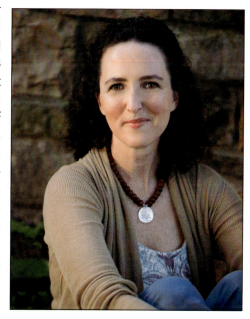

I use yoga asana as an integrative resource in my emotional toolbox. When I learn by doing, rather than by absorbing someone else's words, it penetrates more deeply. So I committed to doing at least one handstand every day for a month. Something about flinging myself upside down and holding myself up—literally—taught me that I could hold myself up figuratively, too. I became braver and felt up to the task of releasing my words into the world and trusting they would be received by those who needed them.

We can also use yogic tools—whether they're postures, breathing exercises, or meditative techniques—in a proactive

EMBRACING THE POTHOLES AND DETOURS OF LIFE

manner to help ease life's bumps and lessen the bruises. As my knowledge of yoga has expanded, so has my ability to assess my own emotional needs. I have more tools at my disposal and have become increasingly adept at utilizing them in ways that help me meet and overcome the difficulties that, inevitably, come my way. It's easy to assume that yogic folks have no challenges because they look so at peace. The truth is, they have just as many struggles as anyone else; they have just learned healthy ways of dealing with them."

Grounded in real-life wisdom, Monette shares from a multifaceted place of love. I may have been anxious to try new things, but I was learning to act on the inspiration I was surrounding myself with. Relax a little. You're growing. Beth Stuart shares from a place of deep peace, a space that reflects her ability to step back and teach from a place outside of her own challenges.

Beth Stuart

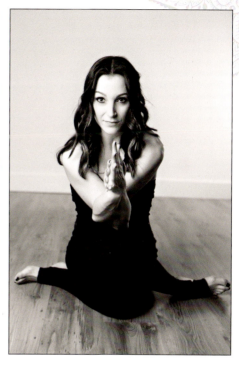

"You always end up exactly where you need to be in life. Everything happens for a reason, no matter how painful life experience can be at times. With the ability to surrender to the things we can't control and move into acceptance of what we are given, there's so much beauty in the journey once we stop resisting.

Yoga isn't just one thing. Yoga is a word that has a vast definition. Yoga is your personal journey—yoga is whatever it needs to be for you. There is something out there to suit all of us. We must just be curious and find it.

Challenge is inevitable, and I try to view it as an opportunity. I've always faced things head-on, dived straight in—even if they were scary. Part of life is the pursuit of continual growth and progression. In yoga, we are faced with challenges every day—sometimes physical, and sometimes mental. I use my time on the mat to face my fears. I believe that we are the most successful at what scares us the most; yoga is a reminder of this.

I have a beautiful young son with autism. The lessons and teachers we are delivered, like my son, are yoga. Yoga is our life. His daily teaching is yoga. He is yoga, and my greatest teacher. He reminds me to be patient, to listen, to connect, and, most important, be present. He is why I teach and is my greatest proof that everything is always as it should be."

We should all be so wise. We can be. Showing up, again and again, builds momentum. When practiced with consistency, yoga takes you on a smooth ride. Yoga enables you to access your natural state, as Sharon Gannon understands: to dwell in union with the divine, a way to access happiness, bliss.

Sharon Gannon

"The purpose of life is to realize who I really am beyond my present body, personality, mind, ego, and unresolved karmas. Through the remembrance of God and being kind to others, self-realization or enlightenment is possible.

The best way to uplift your own life is to do all you can to uplift the lives of others. Contributing to the happiness and liberation of others will eventually but inevitably ensure your own happiness and freedom. Daring to care about the happiness and liberation of others is the most important thing that any human being can do now."

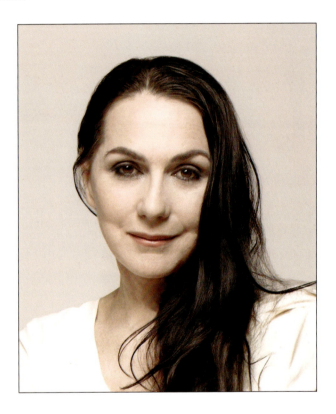

Sharon reminds me to get out of my own way and get into service to others. Once you embrace this idea, other like-minded individuals come into your life. Heather Sheree Titus and I met when she was creating a yoga festival. I reached out and asked her if I could help. As I came to know her well, I learned that she, like all of us, was living yoga, not just practicing poses. By embracing the practice, you can, too.

Heather Sheree Titus

"Yoga did its work on me. Even though I was doing it to relieve stress, the ancient practice of asana will begin to have effects on many levels, whether that's your intention or not. Linking movement to breath with awareness cultivates an ability to be in the present moment that just isn't nurtured or taught in our society. Yoga taught me that I am not my emotions, that I am not a victim of my external world and its flux, but rather, that I am a heart-centered being that can move from a place other than reactivity, that we are not separate. . . . That all is in relationship. Every single one of us has a heart within that has the capacity to shine brightly, and, whether it is shining right now or not, the peace is always there, really just waiting for us to get out of the way and let it reveal itself.

That each of us has a light within that shines brightly, and that the peace is there.

If my world is rocked, which it has been, I turn first to the most practical application to get me through and back to a place of peace, a place from which I can be compassionate and kind, and take the blinders off that may have narrowed my view. Sometimes that's a physical practice—like moving stuck energy from my emotional center with the practice of Agni Sara—transmuting it to healthy power, distributed smoothly. Sometimes it's the ethical guidelines of the Yamas and Niyamas, such as the last Yama: Aparigraha, nonattachment, as a reminder to let it go, to know that change is the only constant. I also interpret this as 'to give freely and to only accept what is freely offered.' This Yama helps to neutralize any tendency to swim upstream, so to speak. . . . Sometimes it's a revitalizing practice full of backbends and heart openers to pick myself back up,

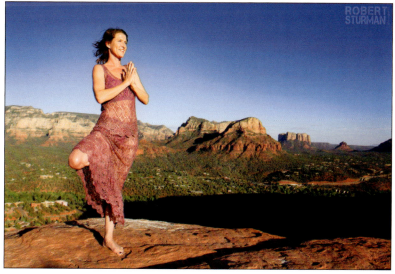

Robert Sturman

or a restorative to remember that I am fully supported and grounded and can relax in faith and trust. Studying the written teachings puts things into perspective, too.

I didn't know how to live before yoga, I don't think. I didn't look inside at all. With a life from that worldview, it all culminated in depression, anxiety, and over-use and abuse of alcohol as trials arose at the peak of life's challenges—the death of several close relatives within a short time span, including my father to cancer, and then my pet, I was forced to reexamine my outlook on life. With no spirituality or religion, I thought everything was random. My own deep suffering was enough to make me look up one day and ask, *What's wrong here?* I couldn't live like that anymore and truly, simply shifted. *Happiness does not come from outside of myself* was the realization. Quite the opposite really—an unending joy is what exists within. I just hadn't seen it."

Out of the muck, a lotus flower grows, just as Heather has seen. I might have thought it was humiliating to have people witness my tears crying out for a sign, but I've come to understand that they witnessed a transformational moment. How beautiful to share our humanity by being open to vulnerability. Often, even if you believe you're an "anxious hot mess" like Jen Vagios believed, you're growing. Jen's yoga practice allowed her to embrace all aspects of her divine light, to see herself as uniquely beautiful—as we all are.

Jen Vagios

"It was a leap of faith, a loss of a job, a bout of depression, and a nudge from my husband that got me to sign up for teacher training.

I started practicing yoga ten-plus years ago. It was a free yoga class offered at a private investment bank twice a week. I managed the fitness center and would jump in the class if I could. I loved the chill vibe of the teacher. She seemed calm and collected all the time, very unlike me: a student in grad school at Columbia University, struggling to ace neuroscience. 'Stress' was my middle name. But I didn't necessarily tap into the spiritual nature of yoga until years later. And now, of course, it's about breathing in moments and letting go of the past or worries of the future.

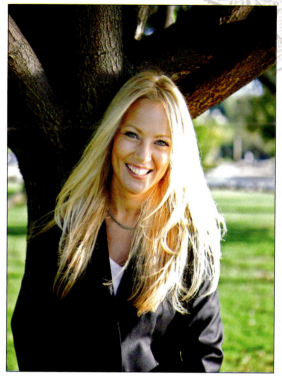

Sometimes I look back and think, *If only I knew about yoga when I was a hot mess of a bitchy, underweight, starved teenager*. But I didn't, and now I know that was my path. Karma. Call it what you may. I believe in that. I believe we all have a path and that we cannot control other people's paths. That part helped me realize that you can't always help someone else; you can only do so much, then you need to let it go. Literally. You can only change your own habits, patterns, reactions, etc.

At one point, I fed into all my imbalances and pushed myself right into hating yoga (let's just say, it was in a room that was inferno-like in temperature), and I thought harder and hotter was better for my fire energy. Hell no, pun intended. Anyway, what I teach now is alignment-based classes that focus on strength, stamina, stretching, breathing, and stress relief. *Being and breathing*. That's where it's at.

Yoga is in the *breath*. You breathe in the chest and you're anxious and stressed, you breathe into the belly (as in use your diaphragm) and you find the *moment*. We are all living in a stressful space most of the time. A stressed-out mind creates a stressed out and uptight body. Uptight bodies create uptight minds.

I can promise, you will start standing taller, breathing, noticing how you react to things, people, personalities, situations, and pause. Your way of seeing things and handling them (e.g., a red light, long line, traffic) without steam coming out of your ears. Instead you say, *Hmmm the freaking Universe is telling me something, like I should chill out and experience something*. Red lights in fact remind us to slow down and *pause*.

Try a class, look for basics if you've never done it before. Leave your ego at the door and step onto a mat: most studios have them. The physical body is probably tight, maybe weak, and sitting still is going to send you into a panic; but trust me, keep showing up, and in a few months, a year, a few years, you'll never leave. It's well worth the first step of getting your yogi toes onto a mat.

For me, yoga has helped me make massive leaps from old habits that left me a bit of a hot anxious mess to a life of more ease, joy, and contentment. Loving my own body instead of bashing it all the time, accepting what is, and being okay with losing control sometimes."

It doesn't take a million years to come to profound levels of understanding about humanity, as Jen has proven. You, too, are a yogi. I try to keep it simple and not take myself so seriously. You are amazing. You have the capacity for greatness. Step into your unique light. Shine bright. As Marianne Williamson said, "Your playing small does not serve the world."

HERE'S WHAT I LEARNED IN THE EARLY DAYS OF MY NEW LIFE:

1. **There is a space between where you want to be and where you are going.** There is an energy there that you can use as momentum for the days when you feel overwhelmed or discouraged. Once you drive past the honeymoon phase of a huge life shift, the second step might take you down the wrong road a time or two, or three. Mistakes are inevitable, so embrace the idea that "perfect" is a toxic word. Simply restart your engine by treating yourself with great kindness, and get back on the road.

2. **Try anything.** Look for markers of courage, because you have more than you ever dreamed of. Smile in the understanding that you can step back at any time, dust yourself off, and start again the next day. The next moment. For me, I developed a list of simple pleasures: audio books with inspiring messages, nature and earth documentaries, and an occasional

massage. Since yoga became more than a way to exercise, I tried new exercise classes at the gym. Yoga was there to dump my sadness on my mat and enjoy the rest of my day at times, but primarily it raised my energy level so much that I had more power to devote to working on my bikini body elsewhere. I tried free salsa classes at dance studios. Surprisingly, it was a safe, fun way to get out and shake my worries away, all in an alcohol-free, healthy environment. No one bothered anyone else, all just came together to dance and have fun and go home. I also did an incredibly scary thing: I took Improv lessons. I highly recommend it. Improv is empowering. It's a great way to get out of your head and dare to redefine what you thought your limits were. Life-transformation isn't intended to torture you; neither should your yoga practice. The breathing techniques I learned in yoga allowed me to face my fears onstage. Although I admit there were sweaty palms more than once or twice, I calmed myself with my breath before the shows. Once onstage, I forgot my fears. I had fun. Imagine that facing your fears, your detours, could produce fun. How would that feel?

3. **Write down your goals: short term and long term.** Develop a strategy for staying excited about them. One of my tendencies was to isolate. I had to force myself to get out of the house and socialize, especially alone. My worst solo trip was to the movies; I left more than once in a puddle of tears. Then, I reframed my outlook. I told myself I was doing research for screenwriting. Working, not drowning my loneliness in a bucket of popcorn alone, enabled me to enjoy the solitude. Concentrate on one or two goals, short term. Reward yourself with a simple gift, like a new book, when you accomplish it/them. Same with your yoga practice. Make yourself accountable for concrete markers that you are getting out of it what you want. If you are bored with a certain style or studio, change. Switching styles and philosophies will guarantee growth. By being open to trying new things, I guarantee you will find new avenues to success.

4. **Create a vision board.** Identify what you want to achieve and get crafty. Find pictures or words that represent the experiences, items, and feelings you wish to attract into your life and paste them onto a piece of paper or poster board. Place it where you can see it daily. Visualize yourself, and how you will feel, already having it. Feel gratitude as you see those things manifesting. Notice how this applies to your yoga practice, too. I once posted a photo a friend took of me learning how to do scorpion pose. Although I had used the wall as a safety net, I was amazed to see just how

close I was to accomplishing my goal. I had become so accustomed to remaining focused on the other aspects of the practice, I had quit trying to achieve a new pose. I'm happy to report that I did finally accomplish my goal of scorpion pose. Remember, your vision board is a work in progress. Nothing written in stone. New goals, new board.

5. **Learn to say no.** Once you know that you want to dedicate a certain amount of time to making yoga a partner for life, you either eliminate certain commitments or carve out time that you don't think you possibly have. Now look at how much time you're dedicating to developing relationships with other people—friends, coworkers, partners, family—and realize that the amount of time that takes can carve into your solo time. It's not good enough to blame others for you not reaching your highest potential. Right now, take out a piece of paper and draw a pie shape. Carve it into pieces and see if there is balance in the areas of your life that are important to you. If one slice is larger than the others, adjust. Keep getting a grip on the amount of time you say *yes* when you don't want to or don't have to. *No* is a great tool to give yourself the gift of time.

6. **Evaluate what your life journey looks like.** Now that you are interpreting how you move through your day, you can control your actions. Just like a yoga pose, you control the amount you relax into a pose or push to your edge. Goals are the same way. Explore that space just at the end of your comfort zone. You are no longer limited. You dictate both your present and your future. As you control your body, mind, and spirit, you become more powerful. Daily yoga practice becomes a healthy partner, which ties your goals to a deeper meaning. Your goals and yoga should excite you. If not, reevaluate. Use your breath, your practice, and mindfulness to examine, daily.

CHAPTER 6

Learning, Changing, and Growing

Looking back, I should have thought things through more carefully. I should have hired my own attorney and planned. I should have hired my own therapist. I should *never* have gone to an addiction treatment center before securing joint custody of my daughters first.

AND THEN REALITY BITES

After signing my divorce papers, I decided I needed to clear my head and formulate a plan to reunite with my daughters. It had been months since I'd seen either of them, and my heart ached. I needed to find a clear way to connect with them in Arizona. Pittsburgh was not a healthy or safe place for me to return to. So I made my way to California to see a friend and just think.

The first day in LA, I arrived back at my hotel only to run into my ex-husband, and another woman, in the lobby. *Of all the gin joints in all the world . . .*

I remained as polite as anyone could be in this awkward situation . . . until I learned that my daughters were there. I lost all sense of composure and ran for the elevator, horrified, as I burst into tears. He shouted that he'd call me.

Back in my room, I experienced something I still can't quite explain. I didn't want to be me. I didn't want to exist. I couldn't breathe or focus. I later learned what I'd had was a panic attack. All I knew: I wanted the pain that engulfed my body to just go away.

Of course, my ex-husband didn't call, so I called him. I wanted to see my daughters. He agreed to allow me—under his supervision. Like a prison guard.

There we were, the four of us, in a public place. Unprepared, my daughters were angry and scared and who knows what else. None of us were equipped with the communication skills the situation demanded, and it ended up being awkward and awful.

I needed a mediator, a therapist, or a friend, for God's sake. Someone on my side who could help me communicate my side of the story. But I had no one.

How in the world could I *fix* everything in five minutes in a coffee shop in LA? *We parted worse off than when we arrived.*

And then, time marched on.

AND BITES AGAIN

Abuse breaks you down to a point of unimaginable blank, bleak vanilla. I believed I'd been very courageous to utter the words, "I want a divorce," but in hindsight, I hadn't planned well. I messed up. I've been paying the price ever since.

Mother's Day continues to be the hardest day of my year. I never know when the tears will come. Sometimes it's on my daughters' birthdays; other times, it happens when I pass someone who looks like one of them or see a mother with her daughter. *I never know.*

I used to creep around on their social media pages. Sometimes it made me feel good to peek into their lives, what they were proud of, and the stuff they posted. Most of the time, it just made me sad. I don't do it that often anymore. Instead, I've learned to give myself love by protecting myself. But sadly, as of publication, it's been nine years since I've spoken to either of them in person.

I did a receive an email from my younger after I was terrified to learn that she happened to be blocks away from the Boston Marathon bombing back in 2013. I was relieved when she answered back that she was okay. That was the last contact with either, despite my continued efforts to reach out to them both through letters, emails, and texts.

KNOCKED DOWN SEVEN TIMES, GET UP EIGHT

I was divorced and elated that my worst nightmare, my ex-husband, was behind me. However, a new nightmare had materialized: my daughters weren't speaking to me. Or for that matter, they were not speaking to anyone from my side of the family. Cousins, aunts, grandparents, no one. I, and anyone I was related to, was erased. I was heartbroken beyond words. So was my family. They all remain concerned, rightfully so, for my daughters' well-being.

But even in the midst of the misery over my daughters, I had many great opportunities in front of me. I just had to take a bold step, and plan. I did—I chose to give myself the life I never had at twenty-four. At forty-seven, I decided to go back to college.

As a result of dropping out of college in my early twenties, I'd always felt like a fraud. By anyone's measure, I was successful. I'd progressed up the career ladder, ultimately to the level of CEO of my own wildly successful publishing company. In addition, I served on numerous charitable boards, statewide. My company helped get my daughters off to a good start, to travel and to meet empowering and engaging women. I felt a great responsibility to set a good example. At the time, I concluded that women hadn't moved the needle forward very much. I didn't want my daughters to face a future that required they be the ones who did all the housework after leaving the office, be the primary caregivers to their children, all the while trying to stay in shape, look good, and create community. It's exhausting just typing all that. Never mind living it. I do hope the next generation creates more equality.

However, I acknowledge my deep insecurities because of my lack of a college education. So much so that, when asked where I went to school, I'd skirt the question by simply replying, "Texas." Most assumed I meant University of Texas. A soul-draining lie by omission. And it always made me feel awful.

Back at college, I took many women's studies classes. It helped me understand things that I had been struggling with, didn't know the whole history of, and how to articulate its impact on myself, my daughters, and society. It also illuminated to me how I could help. It gave me a strong desire to focus the rest of my life on empowering other women. I leveled up my commitment to myself to leave a legacy as an activist and humanist.

In college, I loved how sweet *the kids* were to me. I remain friends with many young women I met in school, who are now scattered around the globe. It doesn't take a psychology degree to understand I received from them what I wasn't getting from my daughters—connection and love. I invited my daughters to my graduation but they never came. Nor did I even get an acknowledgment of my achievement as a *First-Generation College Graduate* (Cum Laude) from them.

DATING 2.0

I couldn't recall the last date I'd been on, but I remembered it felt like hell on Earth even then.

Eventually, I grew so lonely, I joined a Divorce Support Group at a nearby nondenominational church (simply because my Buddhist Temple didn't offer anything of that sort).

One of the few things I had to look forward to each week, going to group felt pathetic. I had no close single friends and wasn't doing well at making any. Full of grief, I'm sure I couldn't have been much fun to be around. Yes, I'd been *doing the work*, but confidence still eluded me.

Eventually, one of my college professors challenged me to try one of those online dating services. I laughed when she suggested it. "No way, only really pitiful people do that." She convinced me, though, that I was living in the dark

LEARNING, CHANGING, AND GROWING   91

ages, telling me that one out of seven (at the time) couples met online. I promised I'd try.

What a process! It took weeks to fill out everything. The hardest part: figuring out my *ideal* partner. First, it looked like everything my ex-husband wasn't. Scratch that one. Second, a list of everything wonderful about my ex-husband when he was twenty-four. All of that, silly thinking. Last, I took a long, deep breath, and went out for a run to consider the wildest thing ever: what in the world did I want in a relationship?

I started writing out the things I found valuable in a partner. This took weeks. And it turned out to be the most life-enhancing part of the process. I realized I was a catch, that I had a lot to offer. For the first time in my life, I knew I brought a lot to the table. No turning back now. I had a girlfriend take a black-and-white photo of me wearing very little makeup and using no fancy retouching or filters. I figured that's how the person I would create a great life with would see me most of the time. I hit *send*.

I took every date seriously. I knew my one great big adventure lay before me, and the man I chose would have to be truly amazing for me to spend the rest of my life with him. Never again would I compromise on what I wanted and needed in life. I was also greatly aware that time is finite; I was approaching fifty, after all. I looked at this next person as the *last person* I was going to be with.

One man was planning our wedding by the third date. He was clearly interested. After years of someone *not* being interested, how intoxicating. Going out with him on my birthday, considering that spending holidays alone became one of the most depressing aspects of being single, it was nice to be celebrated. We'd enjoyed a nice dinner, but coming home, this *nice* man exploded. He said he loved Rush Limbaugh. I replied that he could take me home and we didn't need to go out again. The guy flipped and started yelling and cursing. I was terrified.

One of my biggest triggers is feeling like I don't have a voice. I'd made that mistake in my marriage. When this guy flipped, I argued back, which only fueled the fire. I ordered him to let me out of the car and to never, ever call me again.

The date after that one was my last. I almost didn't click on Michael's picture, because his arms were crossed—as a yogi, body language is important to me. I'm so happy I trusted my intuition and met him anyway.

We arranged to meet at the airport, which was significant, because I'd determined that the person I dated love to travel, too. I sat at the coffee shop, waiting. Five minutes went by, and he wasn't there.

Ten minutes, nothing. Fifteen minutes. . . . Thinking I'd been stood up, I texted him, "I guess something else came up?" He texted right back, "I'm here."

Turns out, there were two coffee shops in that terminal! Confusion thwarted, he walked up, and that was it. Bam. *Love at first sight*. Okay, okay, I know what you're thinking. I didn't believe in it, either. We shook hands, and this handsome six-foot-five man stole my heart. He didn't even have to speak. I just knew.

We sat and talked for two hours. When he left to catch his flight, he asked if I'd go out with him when he got back. I wanted to jump up and down and dance around the coffee shop, but thank goodness, I kept my cool and simply said, "Yes."

As I got into my car, he texted, "My only regret today is that I didn't have that other fifteen minutes with you." Wow. Bam. Done.

Once I got home, after calling my best friend and freaking out, reality set in. *Holy shit*, I thought. *What now? How did you 'do' this dating thing with someone you've just fallen in love with?*

AT THREE MONTHS, HE DUMPED ME

Out of the blue, Michael called and said, "I don't think I can give you what you need and want." So much for love at first sight.

I told him to leave some books he'd borrowed with the concierge service at my condo's office and to never contact me again. When he returned the books, there was a note inside that read, "Don't give up on me."

BACK TO DATING? HELL NO, I WON'T GO!

I decided I'd find a way to be happy all by myself. I was finally the driver, not the passenger. I had clearly shifted from asleep to awake. The application of energy into effort was magical; I felt empowered and effective. The Lonely Warrior was renamed "Spirit." She looked older and wiser—gray-haired and beautiful—atop her white horse. Whole for the first time in my life, and it felt great. I radiated light and love, and it was contagious—people gravitated toward me in a whole new way.

After months of *moving on*, I accidentally pocket-dialed Michael. Working in the Middle East, and 3:00 a.m. local time, yet the first thing he said upon answering was, "Can we talk?"

He told me he'd figured out why he couldn't see me and asked to meet for dinner when he returned to the United States. I said, "Yes." We've been together ever since. My daily experience of Michael is magical. He's more than my dream guy—he's my life partner. Emotionally healthy, wicked smart, sexy, and kind. My greatest supporter. My champion. I can honestly say that "I finally made a healthy choice in a partner."

LEARNING, CHANGING, AND GROWING

Making healthy choices is critical to me now. I've been abused most of my life. Learning how to live in a whole new way requires vigilance and diligence.

I've learned that I deserve a healthy and loving partnership. We all do. Whether or not that's in your life is a choice. The greatest lesson I've learned is that I'm accountable for manifesting all the great things in my life. Yoga has been a huge part of this learning.

SPIRITUAL WARRIOR WISDOM

I was learning, changing, and growing. Concepts like "I am not my feelings, I am the witness to those feelings," as Nico Luce shares, were concepts that were new for me. Diving into understanding new concepts was pivotal to charting a new path. A good way to take hold of your life is to make a clear decision to manage it in a way that manifests high-quality results. If you wish to chart a new course for yourself, get specific about what you want.

Nico Luce

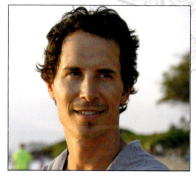

"I firmly believe that we can all be participants in our own destiny by choosing to create the life we want to live. When facing any challenging situation in my life, I know I have choices: I can either open my heart to accept what I cannot change or I can gather courage to change what I cannot accept. By choosing, I am reclaiming my power to create and therefore become a catalyst for transformation. The opposite of that is to spend my time complaining and expecting that something external from me fixes the problem.

We can breathe through anything that happens, no matter how bad it feels. When I was six, my mother died, and that left a wound in my heart that hurt for a long time. I know what it's like to lose that which is most precious, and although at times the pain felt too strong to bear, I learned that bad things have a lot to teach us. Somehow, that experience gave me greater appreciation for those around me, and I became more sensitive and compassionate to the pain of others.

Life is not easy, but so worth living. It has its ups and downs regardless of how much we practice yoga or meditate. Sometimes we feel joy and sometimes we feel pain, some days are easy and others are hard. But when we come to understand that we are not the feeling but the ones who feel, the identification with the current emotion ceases and there is space. The emotion may linger for some time, but since I am not *it*, I don't have to enact the pain or the anger. When we give ourselves space to feel, we can choose an honest response rather than an emotion-fueled reaction. We are not responsible for our feelings; our responsibility relies in how we respond to them.

Yoga has taught me that life and I are one and the same, inseparable. There is no such a thing as *my life* or *your life*, there is only one life, and we are all part of it. What you do to any living being, ultimately, you do to yourself. We are one. That's why we're here: to realize our one-ness. Life is rich and deep, it's the all-encompassing, ever-evolving sum of everything that is, and nothing and nobody is ever excluded. We all must all live to the beat of our own drum and follow our bliss in this life."

Nico empowers from a place of connection to something greater than ourselves. By being inquisitive about where you are emotionally on your mat, you take that wisdom into how you deal with your moments. Speaking of moments, David Magone has embraced the idea of patience, which is the cornerstone of how you deal with your moments.

David Magone

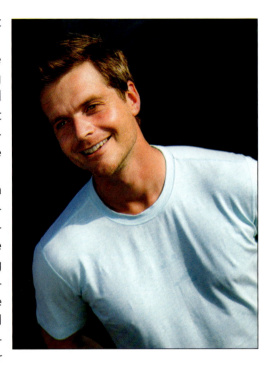

"My yoga practice has taught me a lot about the importance of patience.

For me, challenging situations are almost always accompanied by strong emotional states. Since I usually find that strong emotions make it difficult to see clearly, I usually use my meditation practice to clear my head before attempting to deal with the situation.

For example, when I experience a situation that makes me angry, I've noticed that the anger leads me to hyperfocus on the negative aspects of the experience or person that I'm dealing with. This hyperfocus on negative characteristics makes it very difficult to see anything else. In these circumstances, I find that meditation is very helpful, because it can be used to clear the anger or other emotions that cloud my view.

When I take time out to calm my mind, I find that I can cultivate a more holistic view of the person or the situation that is less one-sided. Ultimately, this helps me understand the situation with more clarity and often leads to insights that lead to a more amenable solution."

When you can step back and see things from a new perspective, as David knows, you can deal with emotionally charged situations from a place that is whole and balanced. While I hear David's message now, I certainly did not understand it yet in that hotel, or that coffee shop. Looking back, what I needed to learn first is what my friend Shelly Prosko professes: being in the moment. I've traveled near and far to connect with mentors like her who could help me to change physically, emotionally, and spiritually.

Shelly Prosko

"Yoga has taught me that it's okay to not be okay.

It has taught me that I can use my breath as the connection to my conscious awareness of the state of my body. It has taught me that I need to love myself and stay present in order to live to my highest potential and therefore love, learn, and serve others.

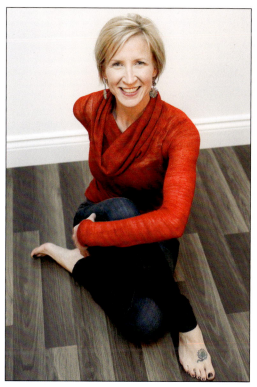

It has taught me that while here in embodied spirit, the physical body is a great tool to use to connect to the energetic and spiritual bodies.

I heighten my awareness to the present moment and try to observe my thoughts, emotions, and physical sensations in the body without judgment or trying to fix them. I try to use pranayama and meditation to do this. I continue to do this, and it helps me stay clear, focused, and present, which then gives rise to making effective decisions that are in line with my true Self and my dharma. Eventually, the challenge or situation changes, and I still try to stay present and simply observe. Letting go and trusting all will unfold as it needs to, if my intentions are pure and if I'm completely present."

Shelly uses yoga to align with what she defines as her true Self and dharma. Once you have established a consistent practice, it all becomes yoga. The rewards of practice, as Dena Samuels shares, is living as your best self—her version of her true Self.

Dena Samuels

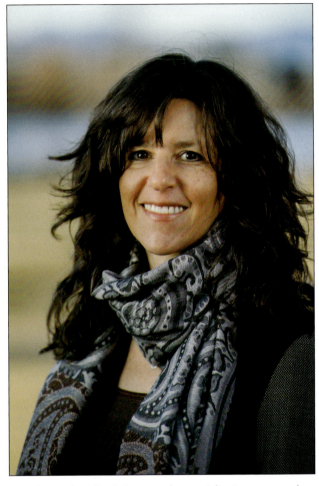

"My yoga journey, like that of so many others, began as a path to healing from the inside out. I am a survivor of severe childhood abuse. As I worked through the trauma of my childhood, yoga was repeatedly recommended to me. When I finally mustered the courage to go to a yoga class, a kindhearted friend took me. Like many others in my situation, I could not get through the whole class. Each time the teacher guided us to another posture, I felt just as I had in my childhood: I had no control over my own body, like I was a puppet on a string doing what I was told. Tears flooded my mat. I left and wouldn't return for a year. Instead, I followed yoga sequences from YouTube videos I found that I liked. As soon as I was able, I found my way to a local studio. I walked in early and pulled the teacher aside. I managed to get out the words that I was a trauma survivor and would not tolerate being touched. The teacher was kind and agreed. I made it through my first class, and since then, I have never turned back. Instead of feeling like a puppet, I began to find the movement of my own body incredibly empowering: a moving meditation, a release, a surrender.

I see yoga as a tool or a framework for understanding our bodies, ourselves, and our purpose in life. It is a means of connecting with our inner/highest selves beyond our selves. For we are all connected, we just move through life unaware most of the time. Yoga and meditation remind us to awaken to that connection.

Yoga is a tool to help us clear out the blocked energy in our bodies. It allows us to clear out the destructive thoughts and emotions that have been stuck in our bodies, sometimes for years. *Yoga provides us a means of ridding ourselves of old, tired baggage we carry around and to feel renewed, alive, and full of hope.*

When I am burdened by a tough decision or a negative thought or emotion, I turn to the mat. I practice asana as a moving meditation. I am able to focus on my physical being, where I am holding my breath, where I am holding tension, and where I can let go. I can focus on the postures, my alignment, how I feel in each posture and through the sequence. Far from simply a distraction from my perceived problems, yoga allows me to put what I'm struggling with on a shelf for an hour or so. I know it will be waiting for me when I'm done, but I also know that when I return to it, it will be with a renewed, refreshed, more peaceful outlook. Oftentimes before a practice, things seem so much worse than they do after a practice.

I am so grateful to have found this tool that works so well for me. Yoga is difficult, challenging, and sometimes I just don't feel like doing it. I also know, however, that it allows me to live my best life."

Your call to step on your mat may not come from being a survivor of trauma, as with Dena, but your call to act is equally courageous. Change is hard, and one secret is learning to let go. We all face and endure challenges, as Mark Shveima knows all too well. He continues to heal and then, from that place, inspires others to move through life's turbulence with grit and grace.

Mark Shveima

"Letting go is necessary for new possibilities to grow.

More and more, I am able to loosen and sometimes outright cut a knot of limitation that has been hindering my ability to do the things I aspire to do. This teaching alone helps me soften in the face of the unknown and more clearly see when I am acting from a place of false truth based on my own fears and stubbornness.

The emphasis yoga places on the breath has been a very practical tool through which one can focus awareness in any challenge, whether on or off the mat. If I am feeling tense or anxious, when I bring my awareness to my breath and consciously breathe for even a few seconds, my skin and muscles soften, my mind settles, and any emotional turmoil I feel begins to calm. I have found that this simple breath awareness practice is a fantastic way to shift my view of the world from an adversarial experience to a neutral one wherein I can more clearly and skillfully act.

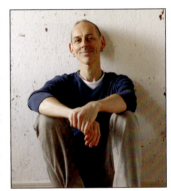

I came to yoga with a body that was reasonably healthy and fit, but a mind and heart that were damaged by challenges in life that I had to face without any resources or tools to help me. I am still healing, but I can act and be in this world with much more ease and contentment while doing so because of the many gifts I have received from yoga."

For Mark, yoga is life, and life is both an experiential practice and a practice of relationship. It is through our experiences that we have the moment-to-moment opportunity to improve our relationships with ourselves, our environment, and others. Through effort we begin to grow, enabling us to experience ourselves as more grounded, spacious, and at home in our own precious life. Relationship skills, or Emotional Intelligence (EI), should be taught in schools. So many people, like myself, were never taught this from our family of origin and ended up with partners who also haven't been taught those healthy skills.

A key aspect of EI is Non-Violent Communication (NVC). I now have skills in NVC. If you've ever experienced what's it's like to struggle in a relationship, NVC is a proven way to enhance your emotional connection to others. Learning the NVC method has enabled Cat McCarthy to have conflict resolution skills. She uses NVC to bridge her yoga practices on and off the mat. Relationships with ourselves and others are enhanced that way.

Cat McCarthy

"There have been two indelible moments when I knew I wanted to teach yoga: after 9/11 in New York City, and Hurricane Katrina in New Orleans. In NYC in 2001, yoga classes were packed with yoginis wondering how to make sense of the event and of life. By hitting the mat, we were able to process as a community and normalize the aftereffects. In 2005, my hometown of NOLA needed more coping tools after such unprecedented devastation, so I went back to help rebuild the yoga community. There was a longing to feel connected, supported, and, most of all, empowered. Yoga classes provided that shared reality and were cheaper than antidepressants. *I turned to yoga to refill my depleted reserve tanks as I nursed myself back to health.*

My yoga practice has taught me to not to take life so personally. To get out of my own way. That my strengths out of balance can become liabilities. That I might not have many options, but I always have a choice of how to respond rather than react, by a simple change of perspective. To see the extraordinary in the ordinary. To cultivate awareness and self-connection, so that I may continue to evolve and become better in relationships with both myself and others. To accept the things that I cannot change and to change the things that I do not accept. To see the nourishment in all challenges, by turning crap into fertile manure. To witness my deeply engrained patterns, discern whether or not they are helpful, and reorganize myself into a new chosen pattern. To receive the gift of embodiment and start each practice from a seat of gratitude. To see living life as an art form.

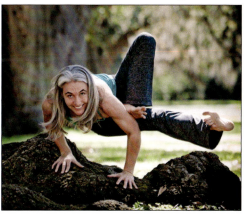

Yoga is a lifestyle, an engagement with the world, and a coalescence of energies. Yoga invites mental dexterity and physical flexibility, while teaching you to be at home in your own skin. You can enrich your life and deepen your sensitivity over decades of practice, never getting bored. It's an empowering and ongoing inside job.

When I need to make a decision about something important, I first step onto my yoga mat. My practice helps clear space, physically, mentally, and emotionally. The more self-connected I am, the more I am able to stay anchored in challenging situations."

Healed, connected, healthy. Cat understands how engaging that can be. The journey of self-inquiry is a lifelong journey. Irene Pappas believes this too. She traded in her frustrations for happiness and found her way to accept herself for who she is.

Irene Pappas

"Yoga has connected me to my true self. For many years, I was unhappy and found it hard to accept and love myself.

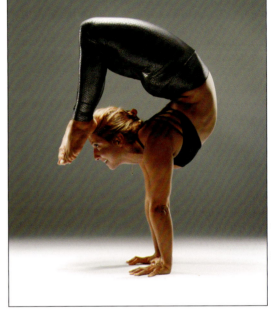

Nestor Villarreal

At first, yoga frustrated me. I wasn't strong or balanced, and I was far too focused on the fancy tricks and poses. As I worked through various injuries, I noticed that my yoga practice is a reflection of my life. When I feel ungrounded, it shows up in my practice. When I am happy and full of love, practice feels easy, my heart is open. I know I am nowhere near the end of the journey to self-discovery, but I am excited to see what comes next.

I use my practice to change my perspective on the challenges I face. I now approach challenges with a calm, clear mind.

Yoga has taught me to love and accept myself, as well as detach from my old habits and negative patterns. I would want to show people that it is possible to find happiness, to create happiness, and yoga is one of the ways to do that."

Irene's practice is giving her a life of health, love, and acceptance. A life of happiness. Dylan Werner will tell you that yoga is for everyone, no matter what your reason, and that everyone can do yoga. He believes and shares this mantra with yogis around the world.

Dylan Werner

"My first introduction to yoga was while I was taking Martial Arts in 2001, but it was a very loose interpretation of asana. A few years later, I was looking to meet girls—not the best reason to go to a yoga class—but it got me in the door. I immediately fell in love with the practice.

Yoga is for *everybody*! Really, everybody. Doesn't matter who you are or what your limitations are, yoga will make your life better.

When I took my teacher training, I had no desire to be a yoga teacher. I already had a career as a firefighter/paramedic and was just doing the training to support my girlfriend. When I started teaching, I realized how much I absolutely loved it, and I knew it was my calling.

Yoga has changed who I am. It taught me that there isn't a difference between my practice on the mat or off the mat. It taught me that we are all connected, we resonate with the same universal vibration. If I can show love to my community, then I can better love myself.

You learn to handle stress, anxiety, failure, ego, exhaustion, etc., while you practice on the mat. When you step off the mat, you are better prepared to handle those types of stress. You can step back and breathe and handle them with grace, humility, and understanding."

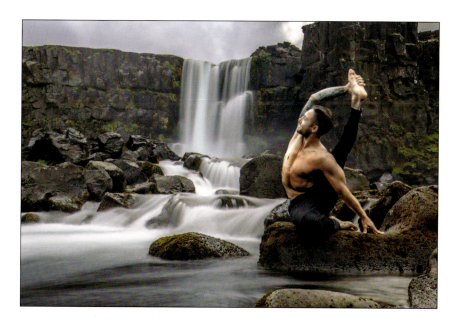

LEARNING, CHANGING, AND GROWING

Dylan is a perfect example of coming to yoga for one thing and leaving with a whole lot more than he expected. What a beautiful surprise. There is no *right way* to practice yoga. There is no one *perfect system* that is right for everyone. There is, though, one unifying practice. The breath. Movement, connected to breath. Being mindful of your breath while moving. All the same language. All shared by teachers who have come to witness the life-changing effects of this ancient system of living. For themselves and their students. When you consistently practice yoga, you have that opportunity, as well.

To chart a new direction for yourself, get specific about what you want. All that you desire is possible for your new course. Here are some ways to help you to change physically, emotionally, mentally, and spiritually:

1. **Physically:** Studies indicate that long-term success is grounded in consistency. Instead of hoping for a quick fix or some magic fad, commit to a mindset that you will show up and move. Daily yoga asana practice will improve your body. Period. End of story. Body image is a separate discussion. Yoga will enable you to appreciate your body for all the great things it does for you. You become comfortable in your skin. Strength increases. Flexibility improves. Blood pressure lowers. Lung capacity and sexual function improve. The list goes on and on. Your takeaway is this: everything improves. This is a no-brainer, people. Grab a friend, sign up for a thirty-day challenge, or write yourself a check you cash at the end of your initial commitment. Hell, treat yourself repeatedly for taking amazing care of the body you're in. It's the only one you've got. Don't take your heart beating without fail for granted. This is your one, fancy, vehicle for movement. Are you beating it up or taking great care of it? Why not love on your super shiny sports car and put premium fuel in it while you're at it, too. Healthy food choices and balanced eating will only enhance your practice. Long-term yoga and a healthy diet will improve your brain function, balance, give you strong bones, and a healthy weight. What you don't use, you lose. Movement is a gift. Imagine how great you will feel at the end of a class; that alone should get you to show up. Oftentimes, getting there is the hardest part. Breathe. Move. Smile.

2. **Emotionally and Mentally:** By discharging tension and stress, your psychological and mental well-being amplifies. It's proven that yoga reduces anxiety and depression. By regulating your stress response system, you relax. In a challenging pose, examine how you react. If you struggle on the mat, are you struggling in challenging situations off the mat? Imagine that you can take this information and enhance your relationships. If you find

you are angry in a certain pose, or about the way the room smells, or where you place your mat when someone takes your favorite spot, are you also angry in areas of your life you can't control? Wouldn't you love to have an ongoing tool to effectively look at your sense of self and community? If you react with grace and compassion to your body as you steady yourself in a challenging pose, you can also do that throughout your day. If you can appreciate all that your body does for you when your internal dialogue is telling you otherwise, you can use that information to appreciate all the unique qualities your body brings to your day. Touch. Ease of movement. Strength. Resiliency. Courage. With time, your concentration improves as you learn to remain present in a pose that you love or hate. With a clear mind, you calm your senses. As you remove the internal chatter, you perform better in all areas of your life. Yoga is a great counter to traumatic experiences, helping people who have been emotionally ravaged.

3. **Spiritually:** yoga is not a religion, but it is a spiritual practice. Your spiritual self can be viewed without the context of the dogma of a religion. For some, you will deepen your relationship with the God of your understanding. One of the most beautiful things is that this deepening awareness will be unique to you. There is no right or wrong way to approach this. With increased spiritual depth through personal soul choices, your ability to live in the moment will allow you to see everything in life as spiritual. You can recharge at a retreat or in nature. By allowing yoga to be a mirror into your life, you also allow it to be a mirror into your soul. Your unprogrammed self is your spiritual self. When you are living at your highest potential, you see that you have control over your destiny. Being aware of this can help you achieve a healthy and happy life where you are dwelling in a place of love. When you are in this state, it allows you to live in harmony, and with those you surround yourself with. When you foster a stronger relationship to your unique self, free from limitations, you will allow spiritual wellness to affect all aspects of your life. You become a spiritual warrior, living with an open heart from a place of confidence and authenticity. For you, my dear warrior, are perfectly beautiful as you are. Yoga only enhances that beauty.

LEARNING, CHANGING, AND GROWING

CHAPTER 7

Making Yoga Your Healthy Life-Changing Tool

One of the life-changing plans I laid down when I arrived in Arizona was taking my yoga practice to the next level, which, for me, meant teacher training. First, though, I had to learn that the yoga world had changed radically from when I'd first rolled out my yoga mat decades earlier.

THOSE WHO TEACH, LEARN

My first yoga teacher in Arizona was Alex. Hmm. Alex. His hair (facial and otherwise) sprouted so quickly, we all thought him a Chia Pet. However, he also had other obvious assets: wisdom and gobs of infectious energy—exactly what I needed.

Though his style was Ashtanga, my first love, Alex's class looked outrageous to me—think mirrors, blaring hip-hop music, and peacock-like students competing for Best in Show. All of which, to my mind, was *so* not yoga. I was a yoga snob, a purist, to say the least. I was accustomed to practicing in a quiet, austere room without mirrors together with yogis in loose-fitting clothing.

The whole experience was loud, colorful, and showy. But through it all, Alex smiled, so I smiled. It was instant yogi love—and time for me to open up my heart and mind and embrace at least an understanding of what yoga had become by way of mainstream appeal. Unfazed by the way in which my new hometown had adopted yoga, I went back the next day. And the next. Ultimately, Alex's class became the most relished part of my day.

Every morning, I had a ritual of sitting on my porch, gazing at the mountains (one, shaped like a heart, could be seen from my bed), drawing an angel card (like tarot, giving insight and peace of mind), meditating on its message, and doing my Morning Pages (three pages of longhand stream-of-consciousness writing, à la Julia Cameron's *The Artist's Way*). Next, I read aloud my positive affirmations. Satisfied that I felt centered, I'd begin my day.

Each day was fueled by the three tools I used to ground myself and bring joy into my heart when visited by the nagging negative self-talk or the perennial longing for my daughters: yoga, eating well, and reading uplifting books. I highly recommend *The Power of Now*, by Eckhart Tolle, anything by Pema Chodron, and Mark Nepo's *The Book of Awakening*.

SPIRITUAL WARRIOR WISDOM

Although I had effective tools I was using in isolation, what I especially needed was human connection. I continued to reach out to the growing list of yoga teachers I was surrounding myself with. "Passionate," "Motivated," and "Willing to do Anything" were my new, healthy labels. If you aspire to have a healthy life, be willing to do anything and everything to make that happen for yourself.

One of the first life-changing teachers I studied with was Aadil Palkhivala. In his wise, loving presence, my breath becomes calm. His loving energy is boundless. Once I began to seek out and find beautiful souls like Aadil, my world began to open to limitless possibilities. I didn't have to go it alone anymore. Give yourself that gift. Discover healers who can guide you on your road. Invite passengers in your car as you cruise along growing, transforming.

Aadil Palkhivala

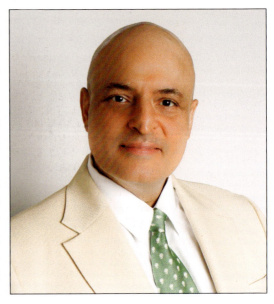

"Yoga has taught me to be totally responsible for all that happens in my life. It has taught me that love is the greatest power of all. *All creatures seek happiness.*

There is no shortcut to happiness. The path to discover it is the path of happiness. Happiness is the road, it is not a goal.

Purna Yoga has taught me that challenges are simply opportunities for growth and progress. Whenever there is a serious challenge, I must look inside myself and see why I invited that into my life. Without total responsibility, there is no accountability, and therefore no hope of overcoming the challenge or learning from it. A challenge is simply a way my soul has chosen to wake me up and help me grow. This creates equanimity of mind that is peaceful because it learns the deeper truth.

Neither I nor anyone else is what you see on the outside. We are deep and powerful beings who simply hold a human form. It is part of the necessity of life to go inside the Heart Center and explore our potential and our source."

Aadil made investigations into accountability a process. I accepted this concept when I finally recognized, while on my journey, that you cannot heal in the same environment where you got sick. *Learn from your new path. Embrace it. Investigate it.*

I don't know about you, but I had put my priorities for myself in the backseat of the car. *No, more like the trunk.*

Before my crash, I know now that while I may have been acting from what I thought was a place of love, professionalism, and spirituality back in Pittsburgh, it was toward others. I hadn't embodied that as personal truths for myself. Integrity, as Melody Moore shares, is built upon presence.

Melody Moore

"The practice has shown me how to be present to the wisdom of the Universe instead of the illusion of separation that I understood, prior to the practice, to be true. Prior to yoga, I was a perfectionist. I was defensive.

Yoga taught me to be present to the wisdom that my soul is connected to a higher source, and that source is within everything and everyone.

Yoga has taught me to stop comparing. To breathe in every moment. To surrender the outcome. To be grateful. To be in integrity.

My body, previously seen as something to criticize for never being beautiful or thin enough, became a temple. My whole life shifted. Yoga taught me to become less judgmental and more forgiving. Yoga taught me to become less perfectionistic and more surrendered. Yoga taught me to become less ashamed and more connected. Yoga taught me to become less fearful and more courageous.

Be where you are. Stop. Take a deep breath. Let it out. Allow yourself to feel what comes up inside of you. What emotions might be there with you, to teach you, right now? Are you feeling anxious, sad, fearful, excited, grateful, happy, enraged, irritated, lonely? Do you even know how you are feeling? Or why it matters?

Most of us are so fearful of our own feelings that we create lives that are too busy and too packed and too full to even allow an emotion to arise within us. This is because we are convinced that feeling something—anything—is somehow going to kill us. We literally feel as though we would not survive the pain of grief or the discomfort of the unknown.

As foreign as this may sound, practicing yoga postures opens space inside of your body and your mind to be able to sense what you are feeling inside of your heart. When you can let yourself hold positions with your body, keeping an even and steady breath, all kinds of emotional responses to those poses will arise. As they do, because your mind is full of trying to follow the teacher's cues to approximate a shape, you are confronted with experiencing your feelings. Even if your feeling is that you just want to get out of the pose because it is difficult, you get to feel that. And, importantly, you get to experience what you do when you feel that something is difficult. Or pleasurable. Or irritating. Or joyful.

This access to what you are feeling when you are feeling it is called presence. Presence is the greatest gift you can give yourself, and one that only you can give to yourself. If you are present to your emotions, you have tapped into a navigation system for your actions. If you are present to watching and witnessing yourself as you feel and as you act on those feelings, you are developing the

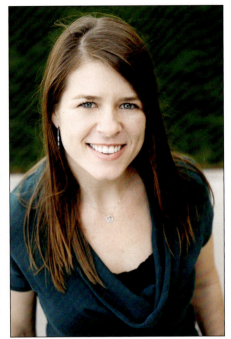

capacity to align those two processes. When you are in alignment, you are in integrity.

The yoga postures that you will be taught will become easier and easier for you as you understand how to be in alignment as you practice each of them. Similarly, because the yoga practice is an analogy for your life, your life itself will become easier as you get in alignment: when you think/feel/do/say the same thing. If you use the yoga practice as a life practice, you can become someone who recognizes that you are enough, that your contribution to the world is necessary, and that you are loved. Try it, and keep trying it, and then try some more. As the yogis say, practice, and all will be revealed to you."

Presence is possible. Yoga is the gateway. Without an ability to stay present to my painful feelings, I escaped by simply checking out. Yoga now gives me the awareness to see when I might be considering taking that dangerous road. I see that signal, like a railroad crossing with flashing lights. I stop, breathe, and experience my feelings. Always easy? Of course not. But healthy. Melissa Smith understands, and shares, why accessing your conscious self brings healthy results.

Melissa Smith

"I discovered that the work and practice of yoga isn't about giving things up or even changing who I am to please myself or someone else. It's a gradual falling away of those things that no longer nourish my heart. All of that seems to come about when I take time to be still, listen, and wait. I consider that my life's purpose: to create an environment through yoga that allows others to see their own beauty.

The reason I practice yoga asana is to deepen awareness of my mind and body on and off the mat. I have discovered a connection to myself that, in all of my ambition in seeking a spiritual or more religious practice, I never awakened fully in my soul.

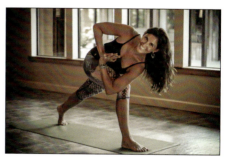

A magical interdependence emerges when movement is combined with breath. Harnessing the power of that breath with movement creates a consciousness that affects the body on the deepest levels of health, emotions, and even in relationships.

Achieving a certain posture doesn't make me a yoga practitioner. Being present and aware, breath by breath, in life does.

Yoga isn't something you just try once. You have to try on different styles and teachers to see what would be the best fit for you. Then, over time, the fit might need adjustments as you transform and change, not only physically, but spiritually. As I've gotten older, yoga has become much less a physical practice for me than a mental and spiritual one. It's my hope that students will allow themselves to explore what makes them feel calm, contented, and renewed—no matter the style or teacher. The perfect fit is what allows you to become more and more true to who you are.

There's something to be said for no longer needing to fill my time to feel special or loved."

I met Anton Mackey in a yoga teacher continuing education workshop. We became teachers around the same time, and were partnered to expand our skills professionally and introspectively. His smile and genuine spirit is infectious.

It's true we live in a world with people we may not align with for many reasons, but I'm reaching out to your sense of choice. As I encourage you to remain open to people with differing viewpoints, value sets, and ways of living, try and cultivate your inner circle of healthy teachers, mentors, peers, partners, and friends. That inner circle you can control.

Anton Mackey

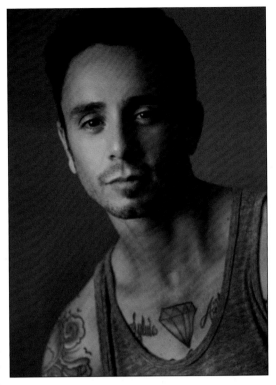

"I believe yoga is a transformational practice that encourages us to look inward to create a deeper connection to our soul, leading to a more healthy and happy life. I love to read about different mystical traditions, religions, and spiritual practices, as well as deepen my understanding of the energetic and anatomical body. My personal spiritual practice is an ever-expanding understanding of myself and my place in this amazing universe.

I like to help students take their practice to the next level through creating a mindful connection to the body, and a spiritual connection to the soul. A challenging blend of feminine flow with masculine power, infused with light-hearted spirituality designed to inspire them to be their highest selves.

Your practice should leave you inspired and full of passion and gratitude for every breath, step, pose, and moment you get to take! Yoga can help you become a better person through becoming more self-aware."

As Anton knows at a deep soul level, understanding yourself is spiritual. As I moved further and further away from using yoga simply as a tool to relax, I allowed my practice to reveal to me dimensions of myself that had been hidden. Kate Connell is a master at using this amazing tool to *live more*. I am reminded, because of Kate, to strive for *true*, *complete*, and *divine*, as well.

Kate Connell

"My yoga practice has taught me to love and accept not only where I am at and who I am, but also to honor the quest of being the truest version of myself through exploration, inquiry, and inspired action. I've used this principle to learn to love my body, to accept difficulties in the relationship with my mother and celebrate the connection, to be present as a compassionate partner, and also to acknowledge my role in cocreating a divine relationship filled with joy and understanding.

It can feel polarizing to be content with what is but also strive to live the fullest, out loud, and complete version of your life—but yoga has taught me how to do just that.

When I started yoga, I thought it would make me skinny. I came to the mat for the physical benefits, but after some time, I realized what attracted me was beyond physicality, and what I was experiencing was beyond my body. Like many, I was drawn to the practice due to the postures and asana, but it became a doorway into the yogic experience and lifestyle.

I hope everyone can find a *yoga* that allows them to dive into self-discovery, get curious about what patterns and habits they keep and free from, and a tool for living life more fully.

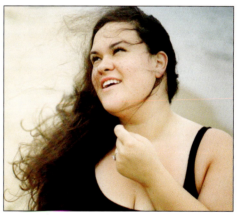

Using yoga as a tool to reflect and then react in the moments where I'm challenged, or a reaction is sparked, the foundation of my practice allows me to have the knowledge and experience to build the tool for use in the moment.

I also use yoga to overcome the challenge of accepting and loving my body, pushing through resistances and honoring my hesitations, learning and relearning to take divine self-care, and to slow the hell down and live life more fully."

What does being true or complete mean to you? Have you defined that for yourself? Recording my intentions, with the prompts from my friends like Kate, helps me do that.

Maria Santoferraro and I share a common passion: blogging about yoga. Maria's passion for all things yoga connects her with people the world over.

MAKING YOGA YOUR HEALTHY LIFE-CHANGING TOOL

Maria Santoferraro

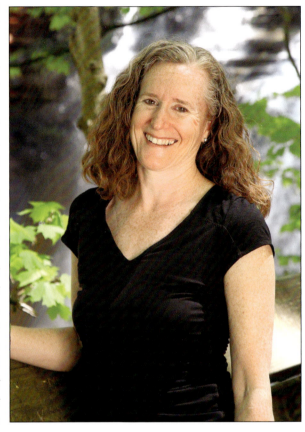

"When we think negatively of ourselves or others, it is out of fear. To combat those thoughts, I have adopted a personal mantra, one developed through my yoga practice: *I Am Love*. As I practice yoga, I breathe in the words 'I Am' with each inhale, and on the exhale, I breathe out the word 'Love.'

Every time my ego mind starts spinning a negative story, or one that is bringing me down, I start to tell myself, *Maria, do not believe that fiction. Let it go, and make up a better story because you are not your fears. You are love.* It is an incredibly powerful mantra, one that has been a game-changer for me. *I am not fear…I am love. I am not judgmental…I am love. I am not hate; I am full of compassion and love.*

The great thing about mantras and yoga breathing is that you can take them with you off the yoga mat and out into the world. Whenever a challenging situation comes my way, you will find me stopping to pause, breathe, and chant my mantra: 'I Am Love.'

Always be a beginner. No matter how long you practice yoga, there are always new things to learn.

Be Present. We all suffer from a serious case of monkey mind: too many inputs, too many to-dos, and too many worries pinging around in our trains of thought. All this chatter distracts us and keeps us from living in the present moment, from living in bliss. I can't tell you the number of times I have used this practice off my mat to be more attentive and better listen to my husband, family, and friends. Life is so much sweeter when you are enjoying the awesomeness of exactly where you are instead of dwelling on the past or fretting about the future.

Let go of attachment. We get attached to a lot of things: outcomes, material goods, cars, relationships, shoes, the past, how balanced we feel in a yoga pose, etc. And I'll be the first to admit that letting go of attachment is not an easy thing to do. Through the teachings of yoga, however, I now have a greater awareness of when I am getting attached to an outcome, and rather than let those future projections fester, I'm enjoying the peace of mind that comes when I simply let it go.

Be of service to find happiness. Whenever I complete a task that is in service to another being, I am at my happiest. *The Yoga Sutras* of Patanjali translated by Sri Swami Satchidananda taught me: 'Forget your selfishness, make others happy, and you will be the happiest person. By seeing others happy, you can't be unhappy. But by making everybody unhappy, you can never be happy yourself. So, at least for your happiness, bring happiness to others.'

Breathe. Your breath can be a powerful tool for stress relief. Next time you're in a stressful situation, instead of running away from it, stop, pause, and take a few deep breaths."

There is no easier path to awareness than your breath. Remind yourself, as Maria reminds me. I, too, even as a yoga teacher, need a reminder. I also have found that being of service brings happiness. I met Rob Schware while volunteering at the Sedona Yoga Festival. I was writing an article on Veterans with PTSD who were using yoga to heal. As a PTSD survivor myself, I was drawn to him because of his work with the Give Back Yoga Foundation and applaud his devotion to the mission of his organization: making yoga available to underserved populations that could most benefit.

Rob Schware

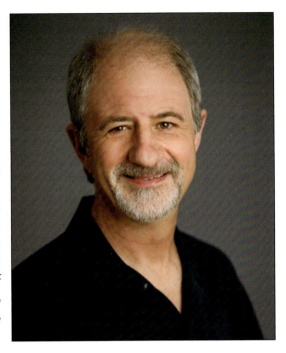

"The mind never automatically becomes calm and clear. It takes work. Practice three-part breathing, explore and notice what's happening with your inhale and your exhale, and then repeat this several times.

In the *Bhagavad Gita*, Chapter 6, Arjuna laments to Krishnait that 'the mind is restless, turbulent, powerful; trying to control it is like trying to tame the wind.' When I am faced with an endless to-do list and an endless cacophony of mind noises, I try to pause into a few moments of quiet awareness instead of trying to restrain the wind as in the above passage."

While on the European leg of my Yoga Road Trip, I practiced and studied with Michelle Jacobi in Paris. As with any studio you walk into in any country, you will always find a friend. I love that about the yoga community. I am always home. In your quest to travel the path to your best self, do you feel like you have a sanctuary wherever you go? If not, there is a place for you. Anywhere, loving teachers lay their mats, ready to serve and connect. To welcome you home. Home to yourself. Home to your best teacher, your own wise, loving self, your intuition, your spiritual self.

Michelle Jacobi

"It's all in the practice and showing up on the mat, and when I could have done a better job, when I slip, or fail, it's only a moment, tomorrow is another day; compassion, mindfulness will lead the way.

If you are interested in making any aspect of your life that much finer, that much lighter, enriching, or successful, a yoga practice will take care of every element of your life. Yoga is your copilot.

I use yoga to access my creativity. Creativity allows me to step outside of the situation and see it in a different light. Creativity throws light on what we can't see."

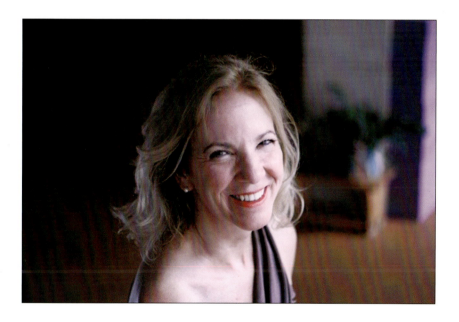

Michelle reminds me that as an artist, writing is also yoga. As a writer, I'm never far from inspiration. Travel affords me great access to my own creative muse. Yoga is the perfect complement to that. No matter what your day job, your calling, your nine-to-five is, yoga can enhance that experience. When not traveling, I'm in and around Southern California, one of the great hotbeds of American yoga. One of the many places I practice is where I found Michael and Amy Caldwell.

Amy Caldwell

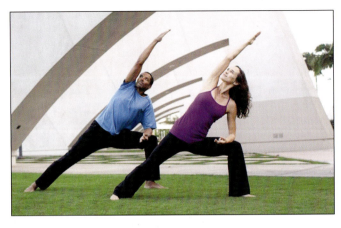

"Yoga taught me that I am capable of doing just about anything that I desire as long as I am fully invested and conscious throughout the process. Like the ocean's tide or our breath, there is an ebb and flow; periods of action and moments of stillness, there is a giving and a taking, and yoga has taught me to recognize that both aspects are part of the greater whole, the yin and the yang, the union that is yoga, the yoking, the becoming one. I can just be or I can do, both are equally valid and necessary. And increasing, little by little, yoga is teaching me that, as Bill Hicks so eloquently stated, 'we are all one consciousness experiencing itself subjectively.'

A regular yoga practice is the process of constantly adding tools to one's metaphorical toolbox. When a distracted driver cuts us off on the freeway, we have at our disposal quick reflexes and deep breaths. When surfing, we have balance, stamina, strength. When we are celebrating with loved ones, we have present moment awareness and are therefore able to maximize the experience and give ourselves wholly to others. *Yoga is a best friend that always accepts and appreciates you for who you are yet still encourages you to be your best self.* Yoga is a best friend with an extensive toolkit.

One breath at a time, observing sensation, acknowledging change, is the only constant. Ebb and flow. When we practice on our mats, we are witness to the process of overcoming challenges. We try to use the same process off the mat."

It's taken a while for me to understand that being invested and conscious keeps me grounded and whole. Guiding my emotions. Faith Hunter talks about how yoga enabled her emotions to be free.

Faith Hunter

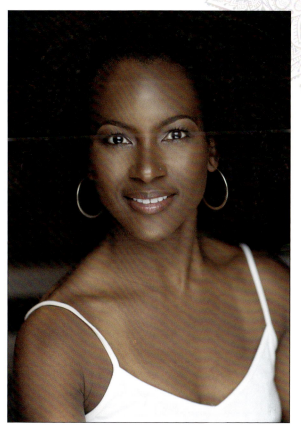

"I started practicing yoga back in the early '90s. I went with a friend as an alternative to our regular exercise routine and as a way to relax. My older brother, Michael, had been battling HIV for years, so I really needed time to heal during his last year and after his death. Yoga was the freedom I needed from the emotional jail I was in. Yoga helped me find balance and joy again.

Start slow, take your time, be open to what comes up, and, of course, breathe. I suggest taking a few different styles of classes to see what works for you. Think about what you need in the practice and select a class or style based on those needs.

Maintain a healthy and active life through yoga, meditate regularly, and you will be inspired to live with a beautiful sense of openness, freedom, and creativity.

Examine and spend time processing how you feel during and after class, and if it helps, journal about your experiences. Who knows what you may discover about the practice of yoga and yourself? Overall, find what feels yummy."

Openness, freedom, and creativity are behaviors that I no longer take for granted. I can thank Faith for showing me just how. Experts will tell you you're born with everything you need. You're accountable to finding it all from the inside out. This is just how Ulrica Norberg views her life.

Ulrica Norberg

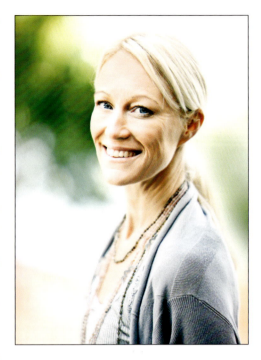

"*Everything I look for, I already have on the inside.* Life is something you connect to when you feel your being side. Life happens and vibrates energy on all levels. To me, life is pure intelligence being manifested in various ways, forms, and shapes.

I have experienced traumas and hardships of different kinds in my life, and in those moments, yoga and meditation have prevented me from falling into utter darkness. The practice has helped to create a space where I have allowed myself to be weak, hurt, and wounded.

My practice is like my best friend; someone I turn to where I can be me and be naked, raw, and transparent. Even though it has been hurtful doing so, I have, thanks to my practice, always landed on my feet afterwards. *My aim is to always try, interact, practice, reflect, and dare to love.*"

My healthiest lifelong partner is yoga. A best friend, as Ulrica believes. The teachings led me to define why I was driven to create this book, my dharma: to inspire people to practice yoga. It's important to look for ways to gain a deeper understanding of who you are so you can know when you are heading toward your goals or veering off the road. Make a conscious choice to bring forth and identify your dharma. Living in dharma means living in one's purpose and expressing it in the world.

Here are some questions to ask yourself to help identify your dharma: How would you live your life differently if there were no limits? Which people do you admire, and why? What were you doing at the time you were most having fun?

We know we are living our dharma when we can't think of anything else we would rather be doing. When you find that you are living from a place of fear or limitation, you are denying the world of your one-of-a-kind gifts. Making yoga your healthy life-changing tool helps yourself, others, and the world.

Many of us have forgotten how to be ourselves. For me, I had worn a mask for so long, I'd forgotten who I was beneath it. It doesn't matter if you haven't attained the success that you want. What matters is that you are engaged in pursing your path. Be a seeker. The path is the journey.

Imagine that you have six months to live. What would you be doing differently? The harder question may be, *Why aren't you*? Can you identify what is holding you back? There's no faster way to get real than to get quiet. Sit down right now and write down three things you would want to hear someone say when giving your eulogy. This isn't a fear-based request; it's a reality check.

Instead of asking yourself, "Why me?" you can examine "Why not me?" If your standard response to a life question like this is to utilize an unhealthy tool like drinking or drugs, you're not alone. Some people simply distract themselves with work or busyness. I numbed out, checked out. Your tool of choice can change. Commit to living with purpose and vision.

The trick is to keep practicing yoga. You can be your own architect of change on the road to your best self. Here are some ways to be the driver:

1. Pay attention to who or what keeps showing up in your life.

2. Dial in to your wisdom, which allows you to trust your insights on your mat.

3. Embrace your unique self, but be aware that the people you admire may just tend to represent greater aspects of you.

4. Connect with a source greater than yourself.

5. Surrender to the idea that your journey isn't always linear. Your calling might not necessarily make sense to anyone else. Make friends with the unknown.

CHAPTER 8

Remaining Accountable

To me, yoga is a way of life—not a practice. A strong, flexible body is the bonus. My practice had helped me cultivate a rich and full life; I wanted to see how other yogis lived it—and leverage their wisdom to inspire those who've never tried it.

WHAT'S GRAY WATER ANYWAY?

I decided to embark on a Great Yoga Road Trip up the West Coast of the United States and into Canada in a rented RV I named Ted. I figured that, living with this beast for a month, it had to have a name. Ted worked. I loved Ted.

First stop: LA. I should have known no self-respecting Angelena would care to have an RV park next to her, so my first night: spent in the middle of nowhere. Ted and I pulled up to the country-kitchen-decorated trailer with an office sign hanging from the shingle, where a retired old proud-to-be-an-American-pin-wearing Gruff Guy checked me in. He was clearly *not* happy when I confessed I'd never backed into a space before.

"Why the hell didn't you get a pull through?" he asked. "What's that?" I replied. With a huge amount of effort, Gruff Guy peeled himself out of his lounge chair and directed me toward my spot. With his help, my first rear pull-up to the plugs and water line was uneventful. Though he never spoke to me again.

It had started to rain, so I pulled on my slicker and, holding an umbrella over the plugs, tried not to electrocute myself as I hooked everything up. Sloshing around in my brand-new wellies, tickled pink to be off on my first-ever solo adventure. I'd read countless tales of lone women travelers (Beryl Markham's *West with the Night* being my favorite), and while an LA RV park is no Africa, it certainly felt like a foreign country.

And then I had my first gray water shower. What's gray water, you ask? Well, it's the bathroom waste that's stored in the RV until you *hook up* at the park and dump it. Dressed in my cutest yoga outfit — my first appointment with a teacher in less than an hour—I yanked the hose out of the slot *way* too fast. *Splosh!* I got soaked. In my defense, the connection was sketchy at best, and it *was* my first time.

Of course, I didn't make the appointment. Everyone knows what LA traffic is like at its best. Since Ted didn't do street parking, I needed to take a cab to the nearest car rental company, pick up a car, and then drive to the studio. And not before I'd managed to erase the gray water stench. I did, however, have a yoga lesson of another kind, by way of a very chatty cab driver who happened to be Indian. Very interested in my trip, he told me he considered "American yoga" a tragic example of fitness—nothing like the "real yoga" he grew up with.

Can't say I could argue against the fact that the mainstreaming of yoga has produced a posse of pose-crazy yogis set on outdoing one another. My hope, I explained, was that, while someone may be driven to my class by a New Year's resolution to get fit or lose weight, they'd come away with a greater sense of calm and an ability to self-regulate via their breath and other sane-making tools. Personally, I told him, I'm all for the social media-loving posers because I believe that any exposure to yoga is positive.

As I drove along the interstates, the cabbie's voice, and my own thoughts, raced through my mind. I kept asking the same three questions: How can I share my love of yoga with as many people as possible? How can I share the beautiful wisdom of the teachers I'm meeting? How can one little yogi make a difference by somehow getting more people on a mat? The result: the book you're holding in your hands.

SPIRITUAL WARRIOR WISDOM

On the road, I practiced with and interviewed yoga teachers and best-selling authors who had already contributed so much to the world. These were my hero's whom I had contacted, made an appointment with, and practiced with before I made the decision on whether or not to include them in this book. I was selective in who I wanted to share with you. One of my favorite authors, Richard Rosen, was as impressive in person as he is on the page. Richard opened my eyes to reframing a currently held belief about how I defined the yoga journey and challenges in life.

Richard Rosen

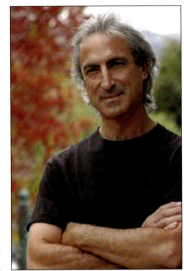

"I don't believe that yoga is a journey at all, in fact calling it a journey seems counterproductive. Journey suggests that we have some place to go, but of course we're already there or here, we just don't know we are, or we know we are but don't experience it directly and forcefully. There is no path and there is no journey; all exists in the ever-present origin.

Life is a seamless whole; breaking it into pieces and asking what this or that is about and what it's taught you reinforces the idea of yourself as a fragmented, alienated being. As Sri Aurobindo said, "All life is yoga," it can't be any other way.

Challenges are living, breathing creatures we've put in place to keep us safe, like guards at the palace gates. When they've outlived their usefulness, they need to be talked to and reassured that all will be well if they let down their guard and retire."

Seeking to continually refine my yoga journey, I discovered Adriene Mishler. Yoga is an ongoing teacher for Adriene, and her definition of a yoga journey includes the responsibility for her own happiness. Happiness is a choice, a do-it-yourself.

Adriene Mishler

"I love that yoga constantly reminds me that ultimately, I am the only one responsible for my own happiness. This is huge. And hard. To take responsibility for your own happiness and to embrace that notion as a practice is yoga—for me.

Yoga keeps me honest. It keeps me open. My yoga has a sense of humor. The asana practice is always asking me to find balance and ease between two opposing forces. It asks me to be alive in the twists and on board with my breath for every turn.

What I experience on the mat assists me off the mat, and what I experience off the mat absolutely fuels me back to practice. It's a great exchange that I give big thanks for each day. Every practice is different, and the practice always seems to know what to serve up. I practice to remain open.

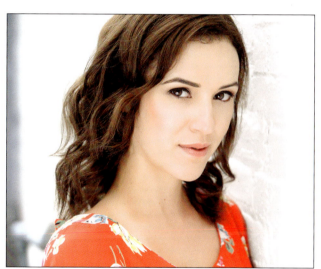

Yoga is really the art of waking up. Getting back to the true you. It can be that simple. Yoga offers up a way to see a world that is working for you instead of against you. Yoga reminds me that everything is connected, so we must live, act, dance, and breathe with awareness. If the journey really is the reward, then by golly I choose to enjoy the journey."

My commitment to self, not unlike Adriene's, is using yoga as my reliable partner for my well-being. All it takes to commit, or recommit, to your well-being is an ongoing support system and a path that rewards determination, courage, and self-love. Adam Hocke's practice keeps him in check, both mentally and emotionally. He is clearly living his truth with steadfast resolve in a balanced, real way.

Adam Hocke

"While yoga is, of course, a practice of union and mental clarification, often my practice drives me straight into my own disunion and neuroses. The challenges of practice confront me with my laziness, lack of discipline, insecurity, and desire for continual affirmation. And I think that's a good thing! I'm generally allergic to classes that ask me to open to Divine grace as a starting point. As I use the discipline and rhythm of practice to calm the mind, I can break through all the messy bits and start awakening to the deeper dimensions of peace and joy that are generally beyond words.

It would be easy to construct a false narrative wherein my original aspirations were all pure and I had plotted a continual upward climb to enlightenment as a teenager. In reality, there were definite times when I cared about sculpting a hot yoga body and rocking a handstand that would bring all the boys to the yard. For a very long time, I clung to yoga's exoticism as a defining part of my identity, a part of my identity that would improve me in some manner or another. These days, unexpectedly, it's becoming less exotic, more ordinary, and just something I do before breakfast to be my best me.

I've come to learn that it is in the pure and simple discipline of consistent practice that one can learn techniques and develop fortitude to face whatever comes with a bit of strength and insight. Of course, we all suffer and cannot

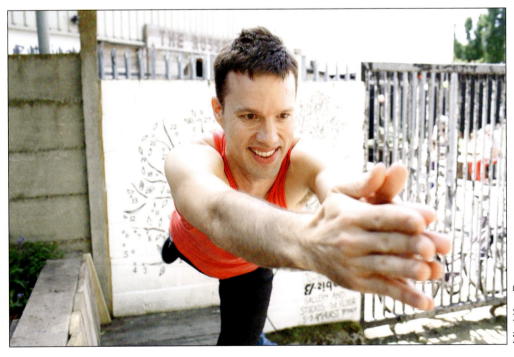

HEALING THE HEART, SOUL, AND BODY

avoid the oft traumatic ups and downs, but the practice helps return me to a baseline where I don't get so easily consumed by my emotions. Studying ancient and modern spiritual texts, as well as practicing and teaching with groups, also helps put everything in perspective by reminding me of our shared universal experience. We are definitely not alone in suffering and struggle. Everything's been felt, experienced, and lived through before. Thankfully, teachers exist to share the learned life lessons, and the yoga community continues to grow, creating so many invaluable resources.

As much as I love attention, I'm trying to learn to step back. I'm in awe of the legacy of teachings of which I am a very modest communicator, and I often stand humbled by the powerful journeys I see in my students' practices. That's what it's really about."

Adam's straightforward style translates into enjoying his daily practice. When you show up, again and again, on your mat, your goals will change. This organic journey is one of the most profound aspects of yoga. Never permit a passion to become stale by allowing yourself to be complacent. On the flip side, though, yoga is not about pushing yourself to some extreme outcome, as Donna Freeman experienced. Yoga is an unfolding gift. Yoga gives you what you need when you need it. It's always there.

Donna Freeman

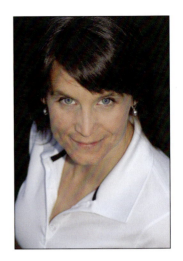

"Yoga has taught me the power of stillness. I'm a very active, driven person, and learning the beauty of quiet has been vital to my physical, mental, and spiritual health. Yoga has gotten me through four pregnancies, a major car crash, training for a marathon, and everyday life. It is always there for me, whether I need a strenuous workout or something to soothe my soul. That to me is the greatest gift of yoga...it meets you where you are at and provides exactly what you need as long as you trust, inquire, and are receptive to the practice."

I'm unfamiliar with any other life science that gives so much by simply being awake. Donna reminds me that sometimes it's simply about being still. I don't know about you, but there have been times when I've pushed for an extreme outcome, only to injure myself in the process. I had to learn how to change my perception about what being still ultimately means to being healthy, as Konstantin Miachin reminds me. To allow and embrace a more natural state.

Konstantin Miachin

"Yoga taught me that I cannot change myself, or life...what I can change is my perception of it, and learn to live in tune with reality and nature." Also, you can change your habits, thought patterns, and so on, and yoga is a great tool for that. To me, yoga is about evolution, love, freedom, and creativity, transcending limitations and not being stuck in a routine.

My favorite saying is 'You cannot do yoga, yoga is your natural state. What you can do are exercises that allow you to raise your awareness up to a level where you will realize and become aware of that.'

As anyone becomes stronger physically, and more stable mentally and emotionally, challenges become easier to overcome. In this way, yoga helps to overcome challenges. Also, once you awaken your creative potential, you look at problems or challenges from multiple angles, and that allows you to overcome them more efficiently."

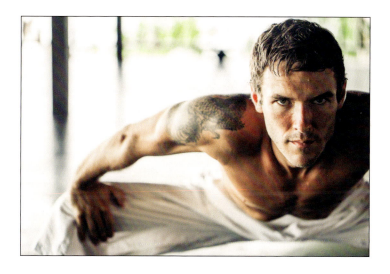

Change is possible. As Konstantin teaches, yoga is about raising your awareness. Self-awareness is one of the greatest gifts you can give yourself. As an experience-based authority, I believe it is one of the single greatest assets you can have. But why stop there? Yoga offers you so much more and can reach into and impact every part of your life, as Justin Kaliszewski knows and teaches.

Justin Kaliszewski

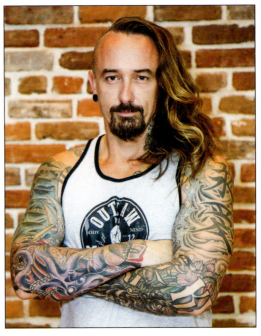

kbenfieldphotography

"Yoga has provided me with a platform from which to examine the self, a method to take a productive look at the past, to build a bold expression in the present. It has crept into every corner and crevice of my life and allowed me to transform my old ways of being—dishonesty, fear, and shame—into new, more productive ones of honesty, fearlessness, and connection.

If I could reach every man, woman, and child, I would tell them that 'It's ok,' that 'We all go through challenges,' that 'You are not alone in your fight.' Yoga has taught me that, though the specifics of the challenge may change from person to person, the tools to overcome it are the same—mindfulness, discipline, boldness, acceptance, and connection. The five foundations of OUTLAW Yoga provide the *only* tool we will ever need to overcome any challenge we will *ever* face."

I draw inspiration from teachers like Justin who have fearless determination. Determination I have, but I continue to hone my fearless skills. I had to own the fact that I was giving fear way too much power in my life. Too many people undervalue what they are and overvalue what they're not. Danell Dwaileebe did at one point, but yoga woke her up to her unique, divine light.

Danell Dwaileebe

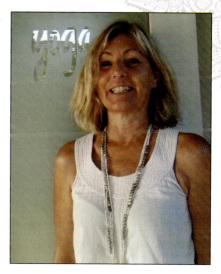

"Yoga taught me (and was a hard pill to swallow, because it felt like ego) that I needed to stop discounting myself. I've learned, as the years have passed, that maybe I do have something to offer—something I didn't know I had. *Yoga woke me up.* The biggest thing it has taught me is to live in awe—the good, the bad, the small, the sad, the smiles, the hugs—and be grateful for the genuine good of others, and to even have gratitude for the not-so-good stuff. One of the most beautiful things yoga has offered up to me is the appreciation I have for being so very present as I sat by both of my parents when they passed from this life. I describe it as *heart-wrenchingly beautiful.*

The more I let go, the easier things are. I use yoga to slow down and really look at what is going on—not what I have conjured up in my head. I use it to breathe—the breath…such a lifesaver. It wakes me up to what is important and what isn't—and what really isn't important, I have learned to let go of. Yoga was a huge aid in raising my children. They went from being a demanding chore with me just trying to get through it to becoming a family that was fun and creative and a joy.

To wake up every day for the rest of your life with your first thought, as you open your eyes, being What? I get another day? Yay! Yoga is everything. Wake up! Wake up to life, to the beauty, to be amazed at the intricacies and the crazy. To look at others as our great teachers of how we want or don't want to live our lives. I wish we had skin that was clear so we could see our insides, too.

It's not about having the best pose, the best car, having the most—but living simply so you find joy in ease."

Danell isn't the only teacher who shared with me that yoga helped them with parenting. Part of my goal, with all the unique people I have gathered, is to give each a contribution that is unique. Many shared that they practice yoga to be a best version of their self so that they can then be a healthy parent, partner, employee, business owner, citizen of the world, you name it. As a consciously healthy human, exposing your children or family members to yoga will make the world a better place.

Think for a moment what a beautiful world this would be if more parents exposed their children to yoga. I'm happy to report that yoga in schools is happening in some cities and is an ongoing discussion in others. I'm hopeful it will be a part of all schools. Until then, you can model good self-care practices by having your children see you dedicating space in your home or in your life for yoga. When you're practicing yoga, your family is absorbing more than just seeing you create the physical postures; they see you breathing, moving, and still in a meditative pose.

I've been at retreats where whole families practice together. Not a mandate for a version of the model family, just a beautiful statement to what is possible. Even if our children only learn mindfulness, or a way to check in with their body, mind, and spirit, then we will have given them a huge gift.

Checking in with yourself, as Charu Rachlis shares, gives you access to your own innate intelligence. Listening, then taking that wisdom into the rest of your day, is at the heart of the practice. Once you've become skilled at trusting the knowledge that is always available simply by practicing yoga, then you can live from a place of equanimity.

Charu Rachlis

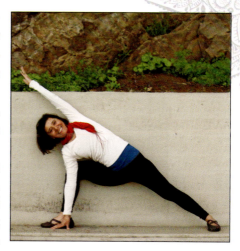

"*Yoga taught me how to express myself—my authentic self.* Expressing from my body's language, authentically communicating what has been my own journey, with my body/mind/emotions.

I learned to be in touch with my body, to listen, to quiet my mind, and to rely on what it was saying to me.

I learned that the body has an amazing intelligence, which I can't control or impose, but instead one that I can slow down and listen to the healing that comes through it and be open to new aspects of myself, be open to changes in all levels of life.

It is a process of learning, a life-long process—each step is so important—starting with the alignments of the postures, how to access the postures, to being conscious and aware of judgments and criticism about myself and others. It is all together!

It taught me that the way I treat myself and others is the way I practice yoga. It showed me that doing a beautiful triangle posture doesn't mean I am free from my dark side. It taught me to look deeper beyond the appearances and to trust this magical process of listening and surrendering. *Yoga taught me acceptance, being in humility! And a beginner's mind!*

Yoga has taught me to be respectful/patient, kind/gentle, to accept my limitations and those of others—yet not to give up, but to learn how to approach each pose with ease and love, so that this attitude is the same with regard to how to live life—respectfully honoring our bodies/hearts as much as possible, so we can honor others fully and completely. *It taught me how to live in peace, inner and outer peace.*"

Innate intelligence works hand in hand with your intuition and through the practice of yoga. Tapping into and listening to my intuition became a handy tool in my toolkit, just like Charu's. Do you listen to yours? It certainly helped me to love all of myself, flaws and all. Loving myself also allowed others to love me for me. But, consistently connecting with healthy souls, like Shayn Almeida, reminds me of the depth in which yoga can help you embrace love.

Shayn Almeida

"Yoga has taught me so much: from how little I know, to our innate and infinite wisdom, from how to breathe and ground and be centered, how to embrace all aspects of my multidimensional self—including the dark scary parts—in order to be a clear channel for source. Yoga has taught me that we are all divine lights, that we are all various aspects of Source: God trying to express itself through us.

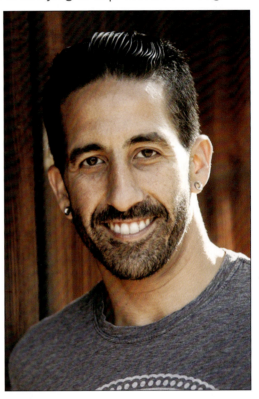

Yoga has taught me that in the end, it's all about love; could you have loved more? Yoga has taught me to open the doors of my heart, to love myself, to allow others to love me, to love everyone as much as I possibly can, and to keep living and acting from a place of love, increasing joy and happiness everywhere I go.

Yoga teaches you to breathe, the importance of the breath and the concept of Ahimsa. The breath allows one to step out of the fight-or-flight fear-based mentality, and Ahimsa should keep us coming from a place of love and nonviolence toward ourselves and others.

I utilize pranayama to calm my nervous system or reenergize my body, I use yogic philosophy to help discern the real from the unreal. Then I try to love more."

The extent to which Shayn has harnessed the importance of breath to deepen his practice is admirable, and it shows in how he sees its value in the world. While love certainly is the answer, it may not be your first response in difficult situations. One way to cultivate loving actions is to start with a peaceful inner core, as Nicolai Bachman has embraced.

Nicolai Bachman

"Yoga has taught me that it is better to cultivate a peaceful inner core and allow that to drive all outer thoughts, words, and actions. Everything around us is changing and impermanent, yet what we do does matter. The best we can do is be positive and caring toward all sentient beings we encounter. Our heart-mind field of consciousness is profoundly affected by whatever we think, say, and do.

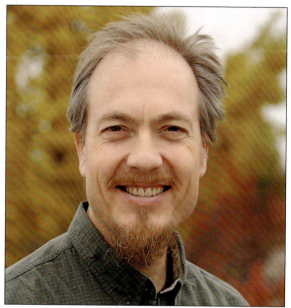

Be an independent thinker and doer, be yourself, and follow your own path. At the same time, stay balanced and avoid going to extremes. When the attention is focused inward, you can be strong enough to resist following the crowd all the time.

When difficulties arise, slow down, take a step back, a deep breath, and contemplate how best to act. After acting, I try and let go of the results, which is very difficult to do."

Earlier, I mentioned refining my yoga journey. Well, being an independent thinker, learning not to listen to labels others place on me, has certainly set me on the path I'm on now, the emotionally healthy path. Is there more to learn? Sure. I'll never stop. Just like Peter Sterios, who knows about the abundance of learning opportunities to change and grow in your practice.

Peter Sterios

"Yoga is a transformational delivery system, helping you live a life fuller than you thought possible.

Yoga creates a state of being, and in that state, challenges are seen for what they truly are, healing opportunities—physically, mentally, and/or emotionally.

There is always more to learn, and life has a way of presenting abundant opportunities for learning. With Grace, you find a teacher who guides you, helping you overcome obstacles until the need for an external teacher drops away and you connect intimately with your own inner teacher."

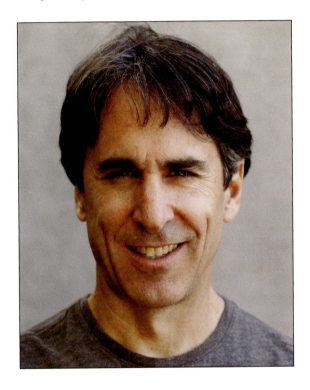

Through the lens of yoga, I've gained clarity of my own physical, mental, and emotional challenges. It's with this clarity that I can address them head-on and step more fully into life itself. Sue Elkind understands this and uses her yoga practice to cultivate her conscious best self, also giving herself a profound understanding of the world around her, and her impact in it.

Sue Elkind

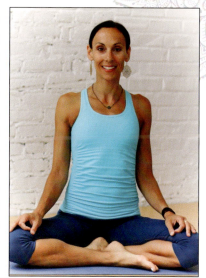

"*Yoga is an invitation to step more fully into life itself.* Every great endeavor requires risk, and in order to make more meaning in life, you must be willing to challenge yourself to grow. This means learning to pay attention and deepen your connections to your body, your thoughts, your feelings, and your interactions with others and this planet. Yoga reminds us how profoundly woven the fabric of this Universe is, and how each of our individual threads contributes to creating the rich and beautiful tapestry of life. It is through this weaving that you can become more skillful at making better choices, at listening and trusting in the authenticity of your voice.

Here, in this blanket of yoga, you are empowered to act on your curiosity and ask questions that expand your experience of what is possible. Yoga teaches you to look for life's meaning in all that you do and helps you cultivate more compassion and understanding in your relationships with others, with yourself, and with Nature.

To practice yoga is to revel in the wonder of the Divine's dynamic play of consciousness pulsating in all things. In partnership with this divine play, you enjoy celebrating the many ways Grace is supporting our lives, beating our hearts, and playing hide-and-seek with us in every breath.

There are no prerequisites or qualifications needed to embark on the yogic journey, only the willingness to show up for yourself as best you can. Yoga invites you to tap into your gifts and 'cook' them into more of their potential. Whether you choose to prepare fine cuisine or just a simple meal is your own choice. Yoga is learning how to take something 'uncooked' in your life and, through the heat of your own efforts, turn it into nourishment for yourself and others.

We all contribute something to this world. Whether we realize it or not, just our being in the world shapes it. Yoga teaches us that we are not separate, isolated beings, but rather part of this expanding, pulsating play of Consciousness that has made everything in the Universe. Learning how to be the best version of *you* not only inspires more people to grow, it evolves this entire cosmic conversation of life."

An ongoing desire to step into our real selves, as Sue reminds us, gives us a place to start from and return to, again and again. I've come to the realization that the dedication to self is an act of love. I am passionate about empowering people and encouraging them to place importance on their yoga practice. My passion is grounded in the belief that yoga is a proven, ancient science of self-love. There was a time I didn't understand what that meant. Now that I understand that, does the journey end? Hardly.

My commitment to my real self isn't always easy. It's much easier to defend and protect the old ways of doing things, because it's comfortable and safe. When you find yourself looking for things, people, or articles to support something you already believe in, think about looking for an opposing idea.

Trade in your desire to only connect with people on your path who only tell you what you want to hear, for having people in your life who also are willing to challenge or educate you. One of the most staggering things about yoga is that it will open you up to the idea that challenges are ultimately gifts, that hearing the truth about your own bullshit will become the greatest thing that ever happened to you. Although it's important to look for ways to build a circle of yummy love for who you are, flaws and all, it is critical to embrace the idea that there are others who are put there to teach you a lesson. Once you discover an ongoing support system, life will continue to happen. My yoga family, this community of love I have given you here, will be there for you. They also will encourage you to grow. Wouldn't you love to become the person you have always dreamed of being? Simply being awake, aware, and true to your authentic self will help you rededicate yourself to living your life to the fullest so you can be that person.

I was asleep. When my heart wanted to support the planet, continue to give to Greenpeace and Planned Parenthood and causes that empower women, the money fueling my fabulous lifestyle was coming from the abuse of Mother Earth: coal. Misogyny of our planet. I sold my soul in an environment that was fueled by toxicity. It was a requirement of the role I bought into, being the wife of a coal baron. We financially supported causes that helped his business. I justified it in my mind because I was helping people live healthy lives with my health and fitness magazine. My actions to support abused women by doing benefits for the Women's Center and Shelter were successful in spreading awareness about domestic abuse of other women, while I was hiding my own. Breaking free from my husband was breaking free from a life of being just bold enough but never as brave and free as the feminist/humanist inside me.

Your reality is created by you. Once you step on your mat, you become a truth seeker; you wake up. Seeking union of your soul and body, you discover a deeper connection to your core values and beliefs and what you deserve in this world. This union, this connection, this yoga requires continued commitment. Make a conscious choice to commit to your best self, daily. Use the wisdom in these pages to support you. Get out your toolkit. Get on your yoga mat. Breathe. Move. See. Act. Be You. Be Free.

Although it is important to love yourself, just as you are in the now, consider that you may be suppressing your true nature to fit in, hide, or keep that social mask on for fear of perceived penalties for being different. I use simple tools to daily check in with myself to make sure I'm remaining authentic and grounded.

Three ideas to add to your toolkit:

1. **Do a daily body, mind, and spirit check-in to remain accountable to yourself.** I do this by finding a quiet place to sit. Close your eyes. Take a long, slow breath, focusing on settling into this ever-present place of support and peace. Notice: What's happening? Now ask yourself: How can I step into my best self today? Listen for the answer. Tune in to your mind. Call to mind a way your mind helps you. Nothing to fix or avoid. Breathe. Check in with your body and emotions. Say thank you for being a part of me. Ask what those parts of yourself need today. Wait till you receive an answer—it might be something as simple as appreciation or compassion. Feel your spiritual self. You are spirit, perfect just as you are. Your body, mind, and spirit are always with you. Ask your whole, grounded spiritual self for a message. Wait for the answer. Take a big breath and bring your awareness back to the room. You are supported. You are loved. Open your eyes. I jot down how I am showing up for myself, as my best self. Ask your spirit for a message anytime. Your body, mind, and spirit are always with you. They are pure love and pure goodness. You spirit is available any time you have questions.

2. **Deepen your authenticity by figuring out a way to get real with yourself.** One of my tricks is to monitor every time I say, "I'm not," or, "I don't," which could mean you "are" or you "do." I've come to believe that what we dislike in others is what is inside ourselves, but we rarely see it. Make a list of the things that family, friends, your partner, children, coworkers, et al., do and/or say that you dislike for a couple of days, and get real with yourself. Do you have the same behaviors? Is that who you want to be? Is there something you might want to work on? There are many online classes that can help. For example: I figured out that I avoid confrontation or, when triggered, blurt out hurtful things without thinking. I did research on Non-Violent Communication (NVC) and have been

REMAINING ACCOUNTABLE 139

practicing new, healthy ways to have courageous conversations. I found out I was missing skills in asking for what I needed and wanted, and that I kept thinking the other person would never give me that anyway. Old baggage tossed to the curb. New behaviors on the way.

3. **Check in with your life goals.** Yikes, don't have any? Never did the vision board from earlier in the book? That's okay. Don't beat yourself up. Maybe it has been a long time since you made some? Why? Get a pen and paper out now and write short- and long-term goals. If you write them down, you have a greater chance of achieving them. Break the short-term goals into obtainable action steps and set realistic timelines to accomplish them. If you committed yourself to trying fifteen minutes of something you want to work on each day, I promise you can achieve great things. Revisit the long-term goals quarterly, to give yourself a pat on the back for the ones that you've accomplished, but also to reevaluate if you want to drop some. There's no shame in failure; in fact, it's the secret of supersuccessful people. They don't fear failure. They find a way around or through a challenge, just as the theme of this book celebrates.

CHAPTER 9

How Yoga Helps You Trust Your Own Inner Compass

My days on the road became routine: locate the studio, get to the class, interview the teacher. I'd emerge high as a kite; I must have appeared quite the groupie to the more exceptional teachers I met on my trip. Most of them were. I'd chosen well; I knew how to source out the real deal. Which, by my definition, is someone possessing skills far superior to the fitness-fanatic-turned-yogi via a weekend certification, who's driven to teach for all the wrong reasons. Sure, I've met self-taught yogis who are old souls possessed of innate compassion and wisdom—but they're rare. My advice is: do your homework. I tell everyone it's kind of like dating: you have to move on when things aren't working for you. I think that's the number one turn-off for people who quit. It probably wasn't the teacher—he or she just wasn't the right *one*.

The postyoga highs acted as a welcome counterbalance to the on-the-road lows; Ted could be quite the pain in the you-know-what to operate. Slow, sluggish, and thirsty—to the tune of $75 per gas stop. Not all RV parks extended Ted and me a warm welcome. One owner, in Washington State, threw us out for unknowingly violating one of her house rules, telling me, "We don't like your kind." Instead of attempting to understand what she meant by this comment, I simply smiled and drove away, hoping the next RV park would have a kinder vibe. At moments like this, breath control came in handy! First, it's not like RV parks are on every corner. Second, during summer on the West Coast, most, if not all, were full.

I finally found a park that would take us in. Granted, it looked like the derelict set of a long-ago-filmed horror flick. I fell asleep thankful to have found a place—and woke to the sound of a stranger banging on my door in the middle of the night. Of course, I didn't open it. I kept a trusty Taser by my side, but still, I wasn't about to take any chances.

At first light, I came to with an emotional hangover that no amount of aspirin could relieve—and the recollection that I'd forgotten to plug my hoses into the park outlets. That's called dry camping—no water, no gray water disposal, no fun.

So, onward to Canada, and the next studio, my head pounding with an emotional hangover that just wouldn't quit. After being pulled over by Highway Patrol and searched, I practiced some of the trip's deepest belly breaths—and reminded myself why I chose to undertake the journey in the first place.

I needed to find a way to lighten things up for myself and not mistake every up-and-down moment for a Greek tragedy. And then the answer came to me: social media.

When I started out on the first trip, social media were just taking off. I realized I could leverage this new platform to get the word out.

I started out by staging reactions from total strangers and posting them online. While filling Ted up at a gas station, I'd ask the nice folks behind the counter if they'd be willing to be in my blog post. The only requirement? They had to say, on camera, "Hey! You're the Yoga Road Trip Girl! We heard about you!" You'd be surprised how friendly and accommodating people are when they know their mugs will be broadcast to thousands of people around the world.

Soon, I had everyone from local coffee house waitresses to big hog bikers bragging about bumping into the Yoga Road Trip Girl. Sharing online became a whole new way to build a healthy community.

WHY NOT OPEN YOUR OWN YOGA STUDIO?

Back home, after parting ways with Ted, I still pondered the same three questions. The solution, I decided: open my own yoga studio. This was before there were tons of studios to choose from; a stand-alone yoga studio was still rare. It seemed like the perfect idea—my tribe would come to *me*! One of the things I loved about owning my own health and fitness business was working with people who were committed to creating positive, vibrant lives. I felt sure the yoga world would be the same. Having already owned a publishing business, I figured owning a yoga studio would be a breeze.

Luckily, I took a part-time job at a local yoga studio to learn all the behind-the-scenes details first. That studio: *awful*. The owners had dubious business practices. They didn't pay their teachers. The vibe: *so* not yoga. I had *no idea* people behaved like that—and got away with it. Inevitably, the studio failed, but I received a great gift. It taught me that I did *not* want to own my own studio.

But I *did* want to share the gift of yoga. So I started teaching at the same nondenominational church that had welcomed me into its Divorce Support

Group when I first moved to Arizona. A perfect way to give back—the church had been there for me during an ugly time in my life, and I *loved* my students.

SPIRITUAL WARRIOR WISDOM

Throughout my road trip, there were many enlightenment moments. Some astonished me with their simplicity, while others gave me pause to think and reflect. But one moment really stands out for me about the trip, and that was the realization that yoga is a gift, and that I am empowered to give the gift of yoga to others. In fact, this is exactly what Margaret Burns Vap shares. Her insights into how practicing a life of yoga can elicit a wide range of emotions solidified for me that yoga is the gift that gives and gives.

Margaret Burns Vap

"A yoga practice is empowering, and healing.

I love that I am able to share the gift of yoga with others through my work; it is immensely rewarding on both a personal and professional level. Yoga has enabled me to meet many people that I would have never otherwise met; it enhances my health and well-being endlessly; the list goes on and on.

Every time you get on your yoga mat has the potential to produce a wide range of emotions. You can end up elated, disappointed, and lots of places in between. But I believe it's the huge potential for our own personal growth that keeps us wanting to come back for more.

Yoga is so appealing because it is cumulative, and because there are connections forged through yoga. Every time I'm on my mat, I connect to something inside myself. Every time I teach or touch someone, we connect. It all adds up. We must never stop connecting.

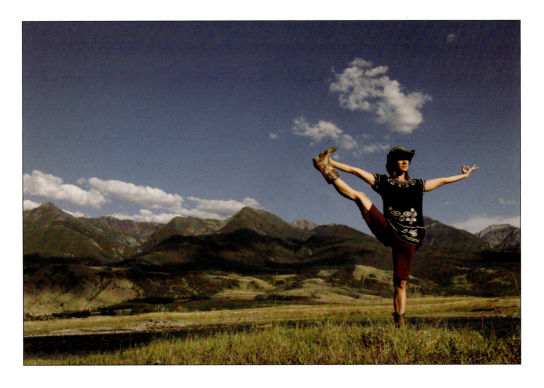

Yoga is not a magic bullet. It requires effort, energy, and dedication. It's one of those things that you get out what you put in, and you have to be willing to take the good with the bad. Some days are going to be a struggle and others you will feel like you could be on the cover of *Yoga Journal*. You're going to have to dig deeper than the surface to uncover the bright shiny stuff. And you're never done. *It is a lifetime commitment. The proof is in the practice.*

A yoga practice can be like a guidebook, and one of its many gifts is perspective. Sometimes, when we want to force a solution to a problem, or resolve a conflict immediately, we can go to our mats and understand that we need time to process. The practice guides this. Through yoga, we can be guided to the best possible outcomes."

Throughout my travels, I've met so many who have asked me how I transformed my life. While the long answer is a lot of hard work, the easier and more succinct answer is that I live a life of yoga. Or, as Margaret will tell you, yoga can be your guidebook. I agree with that suggestion, and I, too, use it as my guide. It brings to me the clarity I need to navigate the day-to-day events of my life. Similar to Christina Tipton, who uses the stillness of yoga to bring clarity into the intentions that guide her life.

Christina Tipton

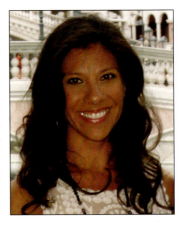

"Stillness brings clarity. Years into my yoga practice, I realized that my curious mind and on-the-go body were often overly energized. My body felt great, but I felt mostly frenetic in general. Yoga taught me to focus on my present breath (in and out) and I began to find clarity. Clarity brings me back to my intentions. Yoga taught me that how we carry out our practice on the mat is most likely how we live, off the mat. When I begin to feel scattered, too busy, and monkey-minded, I breathe, move slow, and practice yoga with the intention to feel grounded, solid, and steady.

Yoga can help bring you back to your subtle body messages. Your gut feeling is actually your body's wisdom speaking to you. With the practice of yoga, we become more in tune with those messages.

I get still and breathe on my yoga mat before moving my body with the intention of finding what feels stuck or lodged in my body. When overwhelm would creep in, I'd identify where I was holding it in and release with intention. When my children were sleeping, during the lonely times at home, I'd get on my mat with a journal nearby, and I'd write. I began noting how my body was feeling before and after moving, flowing, going upside down. I began writing as another form of yoga. Anger, resentment, old domestic traditions were released in my writing and on my yoga mat during my physical practice.

'Be Love' became my mantra many years ago, and I've used the words to remind me to embody (become the spirit of) love over fear in all ways. It helps me to mother more consciously, stay awake to loving-kindness in relationships with others, and to be gentler to myself on and off of the yoga mat."

What we do on our mat is a direct reflection of how we conduct ourselves off our mat. Think about that for just a moment and ask yourself, *Am I true to myself during my practice*? Reflect on the answer, and I encourage you to make the changes necessary to have that answer be *yes*. I assure you, living a life of yoga will grant you so much if that answer is *yes*. It's like Anna Guest-Jelley's perspective that yoga taught her, to be with *what is*.

Anna Guest-Jelley

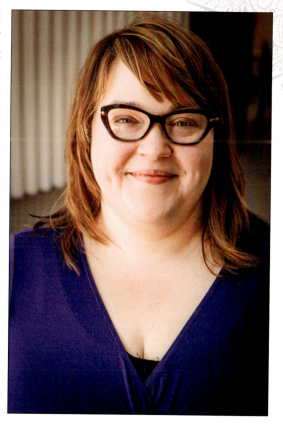

"I found yoga through pain. I had chronic migraines, and I was truly desperate to find anything that would help, no matter how off-the-wall or kooky. And to me, in the late '90s, yoga was exactly that. I didn't know anyone who practiced, and there were no classes available where I lived. But I'd read in a book that yoga might be helpful, so I got a Rodney Yee VHS tape, and the rest is history.

Yoga has taught me to be with what is—whether it's my body, a challenging situation, joyful moments, or really, anything. By teaching me how to connect with my physical body, yoga opened the door to connecting with my thoughts, with my emotions, and with others. I believe it's only from this doorway of connection with body and self that we can come into wholeness.

I've learned through yoga that if I can find some stillness and presence during challenges, I can ultimately find a better way through."

Opening doors and connecting with your inner self? Yeah, yoga does that. I recall a similar revelation on my road trip while I was practicing at a studio after an interview. I wanted so much to figure out where this idea of a road trip was going to lead me when, lo and behold, the idea for creating something to help people just like me came to my brain. While I dismissed it as a passing thought, I will admit, it lingered with me the rest of the trip. Which brings me to the mind. Specifically, the mind and our ego certainly can drive a lot of what and how we do things. Delamay Devi embraces the pulse of this ideal. She brings to the forefront the ideal of how the organic wholesomeness of you can be pushed forward through yoga into making life be what you imagine.

HOW YOGA HELPS YOU TRUST YOUR OWN INNER COMPASS

Delamay Devi

"When life is just not flowing in a way my mind/ego thinks it should, yoga reminds me to have patience. With this patience, I have to wait until the world and/or the situation or the opportunity presents itself in an organic wholesome way, rather than me constantly pushing and pushing to make things happen.

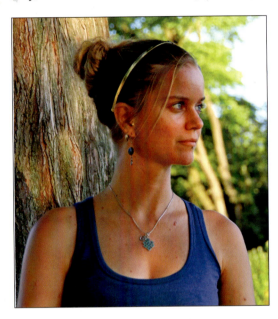

If I am feeling nervous or anxious, I breathe deeper into my belly, firmly plant my feet on the ground, and exhale through my mouth. In doing so, it brings the energy from my head into my body, which enables me to feel grounded and more in control of the situation. When I am at a crossroads, or feeling like I am being pulled in different directions, I unroll my mat and let my intuition guide me through different movements, asanas, stretches, or even into meditation, and at the same time I find I am able to assess the situation and gain some clarity and insight into what would serve me now and not what my ego wants."

I agree wholeheartedly with Delamay's view on patience. It is certainly a learned skill, and something that I constantly focus on improving. Like during my morning journaling routine. I've taken to breathing deep and just being in a quiet peace before I start. It stills my mind. This is yoga.

There is so much that yoga brings to me. I'm constantly learning and deepening my understanding of it all, like making choices. Hemalayaa Behl outlines how her practice allows her to make healthy choices and be more sensitive to her surroundings.

Hemalayaa Behl

"Yoga has taught me to be free and flexible in my body, mind, and spirit, and it's also taught me to be inflexible in certain areas. Contrary to what New Agers say, I believe it is beneficial to be judgmental and have a rigidity in order to choose wisely. For instance, when I started yoga, I was young and going through some trials of life: alcohol, drugs, hanging out in seedy scenes, and partying without any understanding of what these choices were doing to (or for) me. As I practiced yoga and became more sensitive to my surroundings, I realized the effects that those things had on my body, mind, and spirit and started to choose differently. I used "judgment" or, rather, *discernment* (as my friend and teacher Jeffrey Armstrong calls it, from the Vedic knowledge) to choose who I wanted to be surrounded by, taught by, etc. *Yoga taught me how to choose wisely for a conscious course of life.*

Just like we shovel the driveway after a snowy night, we use yoga to shovel and move those things out of our way of experiencing a clear pathway to moving freely in our physical bodies. Yoga is about us experiencing new things, to rid ourselves of the limits that we think we have and go for our dreams in all ways possible!

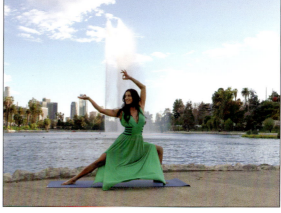
Aaron Dressin

Yoga is a way of life. It's not just postures and physical movements. The traditional purpose of yoga asana was to be in union with the higher power. I use yoga to help me get to prayer and meditation to connect to this higher power, and also my own higher self."

More than postures and poses, yoga is a gateway to the divine. Perhaps as important, as my friend David Robson has come to understand, is the fact that there are no limits or laws to the universe.

David Robson

"My practice has taught me to pay attention. It has helped me to really understand that reality is subjective, and in that sense, it is under our control. I used to think that there were limits and laws to the universe, but lately I'm seeing that these limits are conditioned. No one can be sure why we're here; it's the biggest and most magical mystery.

We are fundamentally independent of our identities; each of us is a point of light, an awareness. The practice is about recognizing and living that truth. You don't need to be or know anything to start.

Absolutely everyone can practice yoga, and everyone will benefit from it. Practice will give us more life, more love, and more pleasure.

I use my practice as a still point to reflect and gain perspective. The daily ritual of my practice helps me to remember that everything is and has always been changing. Suffering comes with attachment, when we need to keep things a certain way. The practice gives me the tools to let go, to be present with change."

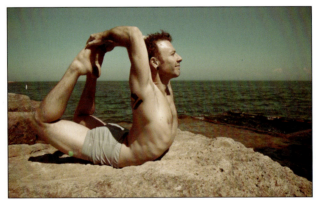

Kendell Macleod

Doug Swenson began studying yoga about ten years before me in Houston, Texas. For both of us, in the late '60s and early '70s, it was incredibly unusual to do yoga in Houston. We didn't care. People were always asking me if I was in a cult. Although I, unlike Doug, was not thrown in jail for doing yoga. You can't make that up. Ask him when you meet him. He, like myself, didn't listen to what his community labeled as usual or unusual. We simply dived in and made it a central part of our lives. I'd say practicing yoga in Houston at that time was one of my boldest attempts at trusting my intuition. I somehow lost that boldness along the way but have since become very adept at ignoring society's judgments.

Doug Swenson

"I was introduced to yoga at age thirteen. Then, when I reached eighteen, I was thrown in jail practicing yoga in Texas. In Southern Texas during the late '60s, society did not view yoga as something progressive and was a bit nervous about its implications.

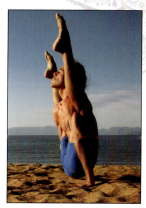

On one particular occasion, my brother, David, and I were just finishing our practice, lying down in savasana (for deep relaxation). We were in the local city park where we often practiced with the soothing touch of nature. As we completed our relaxation and returned to sitting, two police cars drove into the park. The officers approached us. They informed us that several of the neighbors had called in to report two suspicious young men practicing some sort of very strange ritual, right in the city park. Furthermore, the neighbors were afraid to allow their children to play in the park.

The police interrogated us for some time and decided to take us to jail. Partially because we were suspicious, and our answers included the words: yoga, meditation, and enlightenment. We spent the night in jail and reminded ourselves not to speak to the general public about yoga. After that moment, we referred to what we were doing as 'stretching and breathing.' Yoga is an amazing tool to find mental clarity, and I could not believe that society in 1969 was so uneducated—so I decided I should teach.

Yoga has taught me to be flexible in the mind, and to know that all things happen for a reason—whether seemingly good, or bad, there is always something to be learned.

Yoga is not just a thing; yoga is a concept, or tool, to improve every aspect of our life—physically, mentally, and spiritually. *Yoga is your full potential, yoga is your better side, and yoga is conscious living with a free spirit.* Above all, yoga is to find a lifetime in every moment and to really appreciate the beauty of simplicity.

Yoga is too big for one style, Guru, or system . . . yoga is everything and nothing at all, and at the same time, an invisible tonic for humans. I have used yoga to give me strength when I had none, I have used yoga to help me see the cup half full instead of half empty, I have used yoga as my best friend who is always there, and to gain an extreme appreciation for rich moments."

Yoga is an invisible tonic. I do like the way that sounds and believe, like Rama Jyoti Vernon, that it can give you a map of your life. A map that can take you on the most wonderful journey.

Rama Jyoti Vernon

"I never wanted to be a yoga teacher. I did not choose it . . . but it chose me. My motto in life is 'Go where you are invited.'

When I once asked Mr. Iyengar if I should quit teaching because I had never wanted to teach yoga, he replied, 'When you go into a classroom and there are students there, think, *Thank God, I have someone to teach*. One day when you go into the classroom and there's no one there, think, *Thank God, I am free*.'

Yoga gives a map for our lives. Over the years, the breath has been lost in yoga. It is the one most important aspect of the practice of asana, specifically breathing into the back. This allows the pose to evolve organically from the breath and brings the full force and totality of being into the pose.

Asana practiced with the breath is important for strengthening the nerve sheaths, through the central and autonomic nervous systems. This in turn changes the way the brain reacts to stress. The standing poses give the practitioners strength in their own selves, in a variety of situations. There are 84 basic poses and a hundred thousand variations on each. These variations represent all the ways in which the mind expresses itself through the body. If we master a pose, we move to the next variation. When that new variation becomes familiar, we move to the next variation. It is like moving from the known to the unknown, expanding the periphery of consciousness in all situations. This helps overcome fear of new circumstances, giving the practitioner growing flexibility and strength in all poses of life. We have a saying in yoga: 'The way we do the pose is the way we do our life.'"

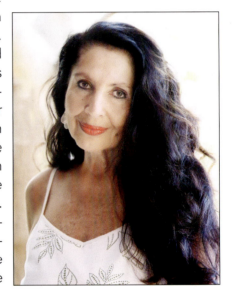

Overcoming the fear of uncertainty was something that I needed to master. My life transformation was nonstop uncertainty. I could have let it paralyze me, or I could embrace it, which I did, and it has allowed me to get to this point in my life.

When I read about Janet Stone's view on choosing yoga, I am reminded of my own calling to become a yoga teacher. For her, it's clear: yoga chose her.

Janet Stone

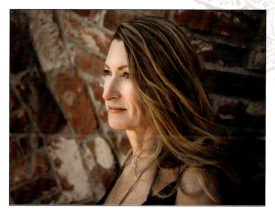

"I didn't choose yoga, but it chose me. I don't feel as if it was a decision so much as a mandate. It showed up and took my hand, my foot, my lungs, my heart and dragged me deep into its seat. If we're to look at the surface experience, I was on a hiatus from my work in the film industry and traveling around the world alone for a year or so when I met a Shivananda baba, and his teachings were the pure embodiment of yoga. I had never felt anything so true. That was the gateway. I still don't know if I wanted to be a yoga teacher. The moment of want never happened. I was completely immersed in another career, and yoga was/is my place of surrender and studentship, and through these strong currents I was pulled down this path of teaching. It has never felt like a want or goal, but the sweetest surrender and a divine offering to the unfolding of my own life.

As for being given the gift of teaching this practice, it's to be fully human in front of all beings, to reveal myself, my strengths and weaknesses, in all places. To allow those near me and sitting before me to accept and embrace themselves entirely in this practice and in their lives.

In a sense, death was my great teacher. My father died at a very young age, and somehow this informed my intensity to be awake while here, alive.

Second by second, the practice of yoga is at the heart of how I am and how I experience the world; it guides me in each action, interaction. Yoga is there through joys, divorce, parenting, death, birth, routine, boredom, excitement, it is there, always offering its most simple and profound teaching; be awake for all of it, the mess, the beauty, bring it all in and include it in the *ananda*, the bliss of living.

Whether I step on a mat, sit on my seat, or have no mat at all, my mind set is on my heart and the union of all parts of my being, obvious and subtle. Life doesn't last long . . . live it, be kind, and embrace your whole self."

How to be a human? I pondered that question after I read Laura Plumb's words of wisdom. She provides strong insights into how yoga can guide your life, if you let it inside.

Laura Plumb

"Yoga is the world's greatest science on how to be a human. It's like the instruction manual of life none of us were born with.

Yoga will teach you everything about yourself—your flaws, imbalances, illusions, as well as your greatness, your power, your phenomenal spirit. It will teach you that you and life are not separate. Above all, yoga will teach you how to love, and in that recognize that nothing is separate. We all belong to life, to one another, and to the whole we call Planet Earth.

Yoga is about finding your heart and figuring out what to do with it. Drop from the busy mind into the quiet of the heart and let life unfold from there. All will be divinely revealed. Trust your breath. It will always take care of you. Let compassion be your way."

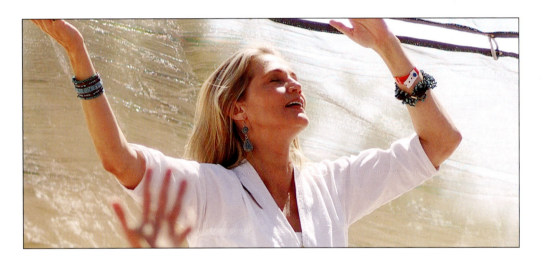

"You're welcome in my class" is something very unique about yoga that every teacher I know embraces. Bethany Eanes embodies that ethos, and she couldn't care less what brings you into the world of yoga, just that you took that step inside.

Bethany Eanes

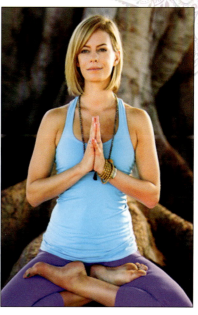

"Whatever it is that brings you to your mat: great! The arms, the ass, the single women, the really sweet yoga pants, I don't care what it is you're seeking. You're welcome in my class.

The most important thing yoga has taught me is that yoga can teach me nothing. Yoga is a practice and a discipline—two things I desperately need. But yoga is not a teacher. *I have to be the teacher*. No experience, on the mat or off, is going to give me any type of enlightenment, any knowledge, any enhancement to my character. As one of my teachers says, 'plenty of a**holes can handstand.' I have to take all the experiences I have and give them some meaning, or I'll just be another a**hole who can handstand. Except I can't really handstand.

You are your own teacher. Yoga helps you deal with the difficult questions and realities of life. All the poses, these are things people do to help them feel good in their bodies. I can geek out with the best of them when it comes to anatomy, alignment, and intelligent sequencing. But at the end of the day, nothing I say as a teacher is more important than your personal, internal experience. Try anything. Try poses, try meditation, try neti pot and mudras and bandhas. When you find something that supports your life force, that brings you even a moment of clarity, make it your practice. And do it. Every day.

Yoga has been the number one tool in my recovery for five years. It became even more essential when, two years ago, I started perimenopause at the age of twenty-nine owing to an autoimmune condition. There are a lot of things I want to give up on, but I can't give up on the idea that happiness, deep peace, and the blessings of self-realization are out there waiting for me to rise up and seize them. I keep going because I would feel like a fraud if I did anything else. Many days, just knowing people are counting on me is what brings me to my mat for meditation."

Awareness with intention is a key to living at your peak potential. A regular routine of mindful breathing allows you to trust your inner compass. Start noticing when your mind wanders off the mat and back into the rest of your day. If you feel like you have become an expert on your mat, you may need to try something new. A teacher will prompt you in the time you are together, but some of the most rewarding insights you will have come after you step off your mat. With practice, you will be open to cultivating a beginner's mind. One of the best things about yoga is that it teaches you something more every time. The successes we have earned cause our mind to become locked on what has worked for us so far. Instead of becoming stagnant in your practice, attempt something different.

Think for a moment about the last time you tried something new. Once, everything was brand new. School. Falling in love. Work. Sex. Microwave popcorn. Texting. First kiss scary? If this ride doesn't seem as predictable as you planned, then you're human. Failure, embarrassment, and rejection are painful. But it's like when your best friend sees you at your worst and still likes you; you breathe a deep sigh. Yoga will allow you to make friends with your most loving partner, your own loving and brilliant voice. If that voice has been critical or scattered, that monkey-mind will disappear, or at least be put in its place—the backseat. No mental chatterbox allowed to drive your car anymore. Tell that mean, false self to sit in the backseat and shut up for the ride. It may try and come out now and again, but show it who's boss. You are.

All manner of things that once loomed large or unattainable might seem scary at first, but your new best self will be willing to suck it up and try, even if you are a bit scared. Self-confidence will build, even if you try it and don't like it. Being bold will imprint you with a sense of self. Sure, it could be trying out that crazy pose you've been too scared to attempt, but it might be something as simple as practicing with your eyes closed once. Or twice. If you aspire to bring a sense of first-time-every-time beginner's mind, you will feel more empowered, like a person who achieves even in the smallest of victories.

It's true: you only get so many years on this amazing planet, so why not make the most of it? You'll be more interesting for trying and failing than never trying at all. What may seem like a detour on your wild new adventure will always bring rewards. You never know what you might find. Peace. Bliss. Happiness.

All that sound too good to be true? Wrong. Even if you have been presented with something new and challenging and said *no*, only to later wish you had said *yes*, you can always break out of old patterns of behavior. You can always take the road less traveled. Once upon a time, I took the easy path. The path of least resistance. I gave up my ability to speak up for myself out of fear. Never again.

Instead of making unconscious choices, be the driver of your own life. Make intentional choices. Those new experiences will keep you on the road to not just mindfulness, but enduring happiness.

Go to that Yoga Samba Dance class for fun. Try yoga and spin. What if you decided to try yoga on a float board? Why not? Or couples' yoga? Be curious. I've found that there are more than enough ways to benefit from a traditional practice. My traditional Ashtanga practice has kept me engaged, passionate, curious, and in awe for almost forty years. Good old traditional yoga may be my favorite go-to, but I've also had a blast wearing wireless headphones in the dark doing a lighthearted class called Disco Yoga. I believe in the middle way. As a certified teacher, I also feel a great need to tell you to exercise caution if someone is combining movement with other things and billing it as yoga when it's not. Dangerous sequencing could be harmful. Remember, there are eight limbs of yoga; the asanas are only a small part of the whole system. Some will argue that no matter what gets someone to yoga, it's all good. I fall on the conservative side because I've had people tell me stories of how they injured themselves in dangerous classes, only to never try another. That causes me great sadness. Our job as teachers is to inspire you to make yoga a part of your life. With so many opportunities now to try, just do it. Try anything and everything. Like dating: you have to go on a lot of dates to see which interests you.

Right now: expand your yoga life. Here are some ideas:

Find a new resource for yoga in your area. Even if you have been happily practicing for some time, search for something new. A new style to try? A new way of practicing, perhaps? Outdoors? A meetup or club? Yoga in a museum? On the beach, seaside cliff, or mountaintop?

Call a friend who has never taken a class and invite them to go with you. Spoiler alert: they'll be thrilled for the invitation. You could even invite a friend to go on a Yoga Road Trip with you. New centers of teaching and immersion open all the time, like 1440 Multiversity in California, which complement some of my favorite life-enhancing centers in the United States, Esalen and Kripalu.

Love to travel globally? Yoga workshop options in exotic locations are endless, and fun. Try a combo festival like a 5K/yoga/music festival. Fly halfway around the globe to practice and sightsee in an organized group, or grab some life-enhancing solo time. If you have never traveled alone, workshops and festivals are an amazing way to start. Meditation, yoga, and writing combination retreats are some of my favorites. It never fails that instant friends will await you. Or stay home and deepen your practice in the comfort of your own home by studying the history or philosophy of yoga online.

HOW YOGA HELPS YOU TRUST YOUR OWN INNER COMPASS

I've had friends sign up for teacher training classes without the intent of becoming a teacher. Try going to two classes in one day. Go on, do it. Be bold. Trust your best teacher, your inner compass, your lifelong healthy guide.

Ask your inner guide if you feel differently after each class. Whether you base your findings on feelings or science, new experiences are creating healthy results, from dopamine to new neurons. Now motivated, your potentially awkward tries at growth bring great rewards. That, in turn, gives you the confidence to then reach even further. If you can, commit to doing yoga every day for thirty days. If you are motivated by group support, post your intention on your social sites. Amazing what happens when you are accountable to writing something down and posting it for the whole world to see.

In our brains, happiness and learning are closely tied together. Successful aging and longevity are built upon patterns of lifelong learning. Every time you roll out your mat, you're rolling out an opportunity to grow. What if you simply decided to believe and do the most unrestrained thing imaginable? Instead of staying comfortable, or your idea of safe, you might find trying that bizarre-looking pose translates into trying that odd-looking healthy green juice you have seen other people guzzling with a smile. The same goes for all manner of things that used to seem strange, daunting, or downright impossible. For me, it was a matter of intention. I made a conscious choice that I wanted to thrive.

There's no faster way to be honest with yourself than on your mat. When you're up against seemingly simple things, like being still or quiet, the bigger things out in the world aren't quite so daunting. You don't want to someday live with regret. The best way to get clear is to try, and if you hate it and it just doesn't resonate with your sensibilities, you can say *no*. Simple as that.

Once you've opened yourself up to a whole new world of wonder, there's no turning around. Sign up for that retreat in that faraway land that sounds like fun. Your practice will deepen, and you can grow in a new environment. Growth begins at the end of your comfort zone. Be curious. Embrace your vulnerability. Writing this book has broken me open more times than I thought was possible. Instead of ignoring that voice inside that kept telling me this book was out of the question, I checked in again and again on my mat with that authentic and kind partner, my loving and wise spiritual self. I have come to know that loving voice intimately because of yoga. You will, too.

158   HEALING THE HEART, SOUL, AND BODY

CHAPTER 10

The Quest for Authenticity, Balance, and Health

I continue to use yoga as daily medicine. I constantly search out new teachers and classes. I consider myself an eternal student. When I go to a new class, I always introduce myself to the teacher. I ask them to watch and adjust me. I rarely tell them I'm a certified teacher until after class. Every time I show up on my mat, I think of it as my first time. Yes, I have a broad knowledge base, but there's always more to learn.

LIVE YOGA IN ALL YOU DO

For me, yoga is about *the other limbs*—the spiritual and philosophical branches. I wish I could say I'm present and grounded all the time, and that it's no longer a struggle to meditate. Or that I don't need the physical postures to access my whole best self. But I do. I meditate when I can't get to my physical practice. No need to stress over which works: both work. Besides, I always look forward to the physical practice. I hope I always will. The more I age, the less I have expectations for the moment to be anything other than what it is. Yoga has given me that gift.

One of the most valuable tools yoga has given me is breath work, which has allowed me to navigate a path through fear and discomfort over and over again. I'd spent decades listening to many people who were living fear-based lives. To be free of the shackles of abuse, yoga taught me to listen to my intuition, even if it beckoned toward things others told me were dangerous—like flying airplanes and scuba diving. I've conquered my fear of the skies; now, time for the ocean.

The first time I plunged my head underwater was scary. As usual, I used my yoga breathing to push through the fear. I'm glad I did. Scuba diving is not a dangerous sport if you follow the rules. While I love to break social and cultural rules, and love life's rule-breakers, I have a healthy respect for safety rules.

Beneath the surface of the water, I discovered a whole other world, filled with life and beauty and peace and calm. The other bonus of being underwater is that the only sound is the calm, steady rhythm of your own breath.

When I surfaced for air, I found myself looking at a whole new horizon. My plans to open my own yoga studio dissolved into dreaming much bigger. I took a deep yoga breath and asked myself, *now what?* I decided to focus on what I've always done—writing. I've been a writer my whole life and finally realized *I* had a story worth telling.

I decided that, until I could find a literary agent and get this book published, I'd focus on my yoga blog and keep going on Yoga Road Trips. I've been on many since, only spending time at home doing public speaking and teaching, rewriting this book, screenwriting, and gathering information for the next trip. Michael is an exceptional travel partner in addition to a life partner. I've met and practiced with hundreds of teachers in over forty countries. As a result, I've become a master of the secrets of the road and will forever be on my Yoga Road Trip.

I thrive in spontaneous movement; new sights, sounds, and experiences. Have you determined for yourself when you thrive? Tons of people don't know, so don't beat yourself up for that one (or anything, for that matter). Figure that out. It's a game changer. How much planning vs. spontaneity? There is the safety factor, for sure. Knowing where I'm supposed to be at a certain time gives me tent poles to use as markers. A mix of planning with room for exploration suits me well, but you will decipher that for yourself. Then there's total wanderlust. I sometimes find lots of peace in knowing *I'll see what I'm supposed to see* in a super-Zen fashion.

Always on my list, no matter where I am in the world, is a ritual of walking into a church where I can light a candle for my grandmother and my daughters. It brings me great peace. I now see this as yoga. Even if I can't find a place of worship to light a candle, I practice an internal daily ritual of Tonglen. Tonglen is Tibetan for "giving and taking" (or sending and receiving) and is found in Tibetan Buddhism. In the practice, I visualize my suffering and the suffering of others on the in-breath and on the out-breath give compassion to all sentient beings. I oftentimes practice this at the end of my private home yoga practice, with my hands in Lotus Mudra, which is said to activate the heart chakra. The practice of intention with the Lotus Mudra is to open yourself to the light and realize that the greatest sense of steadiness in life is an open heart.

SPIRITUAL WARRIOR WISDOM

Everyone can benefit from yoga, and in the face of challenges, you need yoga more than ever. But if you let it, yoga will uncover your divine essence of being. This is essentially living at your best potential. Christi Christensen believes this to be true, too. She'll be the first one to tell you about yoga's intimate connection to who you really are.

Christi Christensen

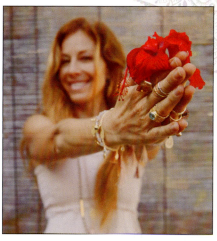

Heather Bonker

"Yoga has helped me develop a more intimate connection with myself on all levels: physically, emotionally, and spiritually. It has taught me about my own unique connection with my spirit and to the infinite. It has taught me to feel, to love, to trust, to accept, and to surrender.

Yoga is way more than a method of exercise. It is one of the only practices that can help every single person who comes to the practice. It does not matter your age, your physical ability, or your emotional or mental state. Whether you are a child, confined to a wheelchair, or a professional athlete, you can benefit from the practice, and it has the ability to transform your life.

Whether your goal is stress reduction, mood stability, increased strength, flexibility, or weight loss, with the right guidance/teacher, all of this and more is possible!

When tough times come up, which of course they will, this is when you need your practice more than ever. Stay on your path. The very nature of this practice is confronting! The deeper you go, the more you learn and rediscover about yourself! It exposes you to yourself, and there is nowhere to hide. But in those moments, that is where true healing is possible. I pull out all my tools (movement, breath, meditation, affirmation, mantra, prayer, writing) to keep the energy moving, to not be afraid to feel, and remember that the only thing we can count on in life is that all things are impermanent, and this too will pass! The times I have been brought to my knees are the times I have awakened, transformed, and grown the most."

The deeper you can let yourself go in your own yoga practice, the more you will discover about yourself. Who wouldn't want that? As my own journey unfolds, I too have discovered how not to be afraid to feel. Your practice also has the infinite ability to show you a new way of thinking—that is, of course, if you let it. Drew Osborne knows just how to let his practice show him a new and different way to look at himself from the inside out.

THE QUEST FOR AUTHENTICITY, BALANCE, AND HEALTH

Drew Osborne

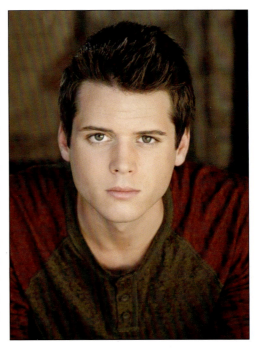

"Yoga has taught me a new way of thinking. Yoga has taught me to love my body and mind but that I am not either of them. It has connected me to my true self and allowed me to observe this life and understand the gift that it is. It has taught me the beauty of community. It has given me the ability to love.

Ignore the misconceptions and stop the excuses. 'I'm not flexible,' 'I want a real workout,' blah, blah, blah. Yoga is for anyone and everyone.

On top of that, bringing awareness to the fact that yoga doesn't mean you have to convert to some new ideology or religion. It is a safe haven, and a place to work on the self. It's whatever you want it to be, for you."

I remember when I first started my practice in Texas, it was considered extremely unusual, steeped in ideology and misinterpreted as a religion. As Drew points out, that couldn't be any further from the truth. I do admire his simple truth: "It's what you want it to be, as long as it's for you." Erika Burkhalter carries a similar ethos with her. She has used yoga as a means to survive, both spiritually and physically, through the ebb and flow of her life. *Yoga is an active practice of being in the solution.*

Erika Burkhalter

"When I was twenty, I was run over by a truck and was not expected to survive. I did survive, and I used yoga to bring mobility back into my body.

Then, when I was thirty-eight, I came down with a very rare autoimmune disease called Guillain–Barré syndrome. It is normally a one-time thing that reverses itself for the most part, but it manifests like MS. The body attacks the myelin sheaths around the nerves, and you lose sensation and become increasingly paralyzed. I had a moderate case. My yoga practice went from working on the third series to barely being able to walk and losing sensation over most of my body and only being able to do restorative poses. In my recovery, I realized how important it was to put your body through a range of movements and challenges. Doing a set practice every day can build a lot of strength, but in order to regain a full range of movement and strength, I needed to really focus on a diversified flow practice.

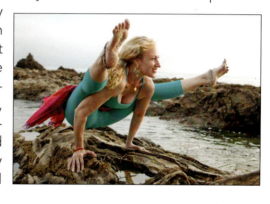

And it worked. My recovery was very good. I still have a little numbness in my feet and some nerve issues when it gets cold, but I don't think most people would ever really know that by watching me practice. The big lesson for me, though, was that it is good to be challenged in new ways, and what helped me in my recovery was probably very helpful to yoga practitioners of all types.

There is an old story about a seeker looking for enlightenment, and when he finds his guru, the guru overfills the seeker's cup of tea while the seeker is caught up in telling the guru about his path. This act symbolizes the seeker's inability to receive new teachings because he is already 'filled to the brim' with what he thinks he needs. We need to always be open and receptive to what the Universe wants to tell us.

Yoga is for everybody. It is a mind-body practice with a multitude of forms that can be adapted for anybody."

Yoga is, by definition, universally adaptable to you and whatever life condition you find yourself involved with. I know Jay Fields uses her practice to reground herself in the reality of what her body says, not what her mind thinks. Use your yoga practice to move out of your head and into your heart.

Jay Fields

"I use yoga to help me loosen my mind's grip on the world and to come back to reality through my body. A bumper sticker I saw for the first time today said: 'Reality: it's not what you think!' So true!

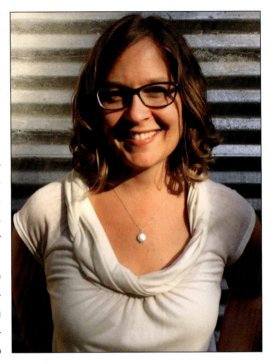

I'm a thinker. I have spent my life thinking about things, analyzing, explaining, trying to make meaning—rather than simply being in an experience. Almost all the challenges I've faced in my life have in some way to do with my mind being in resistance or reaction to some experience that I don't want to feel. Yoga helps me to come back to my body. To feel. To become embodied again so that I can not only be in touch with what's actually real in any given moment, but also in touch with my inner resources.

Neuroscience research shows that when a person has embodied self-awareness, they have access to greater intuition and compassion, more capacity to quell fear and to manage emotions, and increased empathy and attunement with others. Essentially, all the qualities a human being needs to be resilient, to overcome challenges, and to be the best version of themselves. So, in that way, the practice of yoga gives me a good shot at being the most integrated, most resourced, and best version of myself."

I've worked very hard at embracing the behavior of nonjudgmental awareness. I won't say it's easy, and I do catch myself from time to time, but my practice gives me the strength I need. But more to this idea, Annie Carpenter points out that a yoga practice is a pathway to building this awareness as well as practicing patience and compassion.

Annie Carpenter

"Like so many teenagers in the late '60s and '70s, I was experimenting with drugs. Luckily, my mom saw it and steered me to an afterschool program for drug abusers that offered yoga. It was an easy choice to let go of drugging and tune into the joys of the present moment.

Everyone has their own practice. Even in a group setting, each yogi is constantly invited to observe and make choices about how the practice is shaped for him or her. If this aspect of yoga is encouraged from the start, I think the great gifts of yoga are assimilated sooner: build nonjudgmental awareness; practice patience, compassion, and kindness; we are all the same (one).

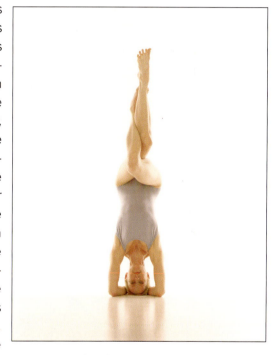

Yoga teaches us that although it's easy to see a challenge—like pain—as one giant, overwhelming event, it's not really like that. As we learn to perceive things moment to moment—in this case, sensation by sensation—we find that we can deal with the smaller, momentary, less intense events one by one as they arise and, indeed, inevitably pass away. Even as they are followed by another intense event or sensation, we can manage them one by one. And we are buoyed by each small success and, of course, by the knowledge that others in our community are riding the same waves as we are. Over time, the deeper insights begin to arrive: that all the challenges, including pain, are happening in the phenomenological, material world that is constantly changing; and we are infinitely eased through challenges when we are able to also know that there is something lasting and nonchanging, spirit."

I've learned to be observant in staying accountable to myself for designing my own life, and the thing I can control is me and my emotions. Everything else, I can't. Nor do I want to. The way in which I harmonize this principle is through yoga—much like how Jennifer Williams-Fields approaches her practice. Yoga enabled her to find the answers she needed.

Jennifer Williams-Fields

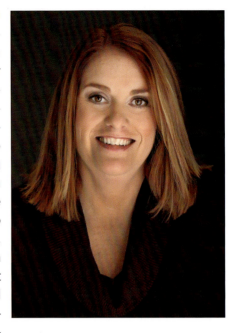

"Yoga taught me that I know nothing, and I have no power to control everything and everyone around me! I've learned that all I can do, in fact, all I am supposed to do, is center myself, calm myself, and allow my life to unfold. I spent many years reacting to situations in my life: a bad marriage, a messy divorce, the death of my mother. I tried to muscle my way through situations, forcing what I thought was best for everyone on those around me. It didn't work. I became more upset and unhappy. Once I learned to take a step back and check in with myself, then I could better respond to my life in a healthier, more productive way. I learned it is better to respond than to react. In yoga, I teach my students to not worry what is happening on somebody else's mat; stay focused only on how you feel on your mat. In life, when I take care of myself and pay attention to my own needs, I'm so much better able to help and take care of those around me.

I believe all our bodies crave movement. Yoga has made me more in tune with what my body is telling me. I'm now acutely aware that my struggle with depression is helped immensely by exercise.

There will be challenges and disappointments in life. Yoga helps me to stay calm while the storm is brewing, and to see the beauty after the storm passes.

I'm a mom and a yoga teacher. I don't have all the answers. I have been fortunate to find a path that helped me seek the answers I so desperately needed. I am immensely grateful to the teachers that came into my life exactly at the times I needed them. I know I will falter and fail. But I have learned the real lesson is in getting back up, gaining wisdom from the experience, and moving on."

What will you do when a crack in consciousness changes your world in a matter of minutes? Nothing can prepare you for catastrophic events. But what about after? What if breathing, meditation, and yoga could soften the inevitable blow? This is the idea behind how Iara Judelle embraces yoga and uses it to move through whatever binds her.

Tara Judelle

"I had been practicing yoga for four years and was a writer/director living in Los Angeles. I whimsically named the production company Kali Films. Kali is the fierce goddess who exists to cut away all falsehoods and ego structures that bind. Twenty-three days into filming, arsonists set fire to our main set.

I was a director with a lot of money and the mantra *no one can tell me no*. The fire illuminated for me my attachment to my identity and my ego but ultimately set me on my right path. I wouldn't realize that for years, but it let me know that the story of our lives contains many clues and ironies that, if we start to pay close attention, we will see all the time.

So after a year of making my own independent film, and many things going wrong in that process, I decided to take teacher's training in order to get back into my practice. *The first week of the training was 9/11/2001.*

When that crack in consciousness changed the world in minutes, my entire body/mind changed. I knew at the end of my life I won't want my struggle with making films, or even the contribution they may or may not have, to be my life. I wanted a life that was dedicated to helping others in an authentic way. Since that training, I have never stopped teaching yoga. *In truth, everything is yoga.*

Yoga is so much more than asana. Whether you want to call it Brahman, Buddha mind, unified field, or God—yoga is about the remembrance of what we always already have been.

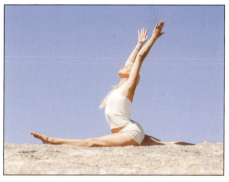
Gina Cholick

If yoga is the practice of ridding ourselves of that which binds, I use whatever tools I have to address the challenge. Often, meditation resets my mind into a vast clarity and possibility that absorbs limited thoughts. Asana helps to restore my body in the same way. Reading texts reminds me of the play of consciousness, and how the instrument of the mind can either bind or free. I use the combination to constantly see how I can address whatever is in front of me from the most illuminating angle. I catch myself when my small self is dominating and work to see which tool can bring me back to my higher self."

Yoga can help you reignite and rethink how you look at the world. As Kim Shand explains, yoga can help you rethink how you navigate your challenges, big and small, physical and emotional.

Kim Shand

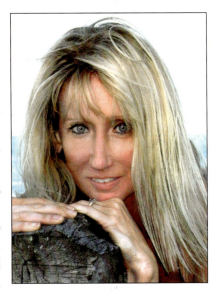

"I started yoga when I was very young, to overcome a spinal birth defect that doctors believed would paralyze me. At that point, my practice was almost entirely about the physical. I discovered my body's ability to heal, change, and recreate itself when it's not restricted by the limits of my, and others', belief systems. About fifteen years ago, I went through a few years that felt as though life had thrown down the gauntlet and I had lost. A series of losses and obstacles left me feeling weak, vulnerable, and spiritually ungrounded. I came back to yoga in search of a different type of remedy, and, again, I discovered that I am resilient and capable of healing. Challenges, dark times, and shadow emotions are part of our journey and part of the gift of being human. When we learn how to receive the gifts that our difficulties offer, we gain a strength that's well beyond the strength of our biceps. Our real strength, opportunity, and potential lie in our ability to fully engage life again and again.

We all have the birthright and the capacity to realize a life of joy, meaning, and purpose. We can be more, do more, and control more of our lives than we think. We go through periods, especially as we age, when we no longer believe we can build muscle, or build influence or satisfaction, so we stop trying. We think constant pain is common and develop a *fear of failure* that prevents us from pursuing risks or taking on new adventures. As our lives and bodies change, we give up our sense of power along with our skinny jeans. It happens because we lie to ourselves that we can't look good, feel good, or be sexy. I believe we all have what it takes to be healthy, to live vibrantly, and with great passion. There is a light inside of each of us that too often goes dim. *No matter where you are in life, you can reignite and rethink yourself.*"

Not only does yoga have the ability to help you, but you can use it to help others just by practicing. Sari Leigh had this epiphany at an early time in her life and has used it as a guiding light on her journey to helping others in her community.

Sari Leigh

"I realized that I needed to become a yoga teacher one morning while riding a bus from my neighborhood in Anacostia, Washington, D.C., toward my graduate class at The George Washington University in Foggy Bottom. I had recently returned from a week of eating vegan gourmet cuisine at a posh yoga resort. Yet here in my neighborhood of Anacostia, none of my experiences mattered. At the time, my personal yoga journey had no impact on how women in Anacostia were caring for themselves and their families. I knew that Anacostia was less than five miles from the White House, yet it was one of the most neglected neighborhoods in Washington, D.C. There were no places to buy fresh foods, no safe spaces to exercise for women, and no political will to focus on health. I wanted to do something to change all of these things. So I decided to use the most powerful resource available to me: my knowledge of yoga.

Yoga alone has not taught me anything about myself. Rather, the people whom I have met as a result of practicing yoga have helped me to better understand yoga. The beautiful thing about yoga is that the word itself translates to 'union.'

Yoga taught me to see the life in people who couldn't move through life in the same way. Yoga reminded me that there are limitations in the physical body yet no limitations in the spirit. I learned to view the asana practice as a component of yoga also, helping me to see our physical bodies as just one element of our lives. This awakening taught me to experience inner and outer awareness in

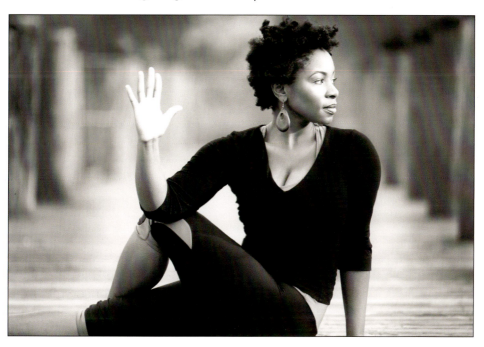

a yoga practice. Yoga taught me to see breath, spirit, and life in spaces of stillness.

We have the tools within us to manage life's up and downs. Every living thing on the planet deals with stress. However, every living thing has adapted to manage the stress. Human beings are no different.

Yoga is one of the most sophisticated systems in the history of mind-body spirituality. Yet it is also one of the most accessible forms of self-healing.

There are three critical tools that I use when I am faced with challenges. The first is to ask myself, 'How should I respond?' This helps me become aware of where I am and gain clarity on what is really going on. The second tool is to take fifteen seconds to breathe. This is especially effective if I am in a challenge and I don't have much time to think. Inhaling for seven seconds helps me take in the situation. Holding the breath for one second helps my mind to clear the slate, and exhaling for seven seconds allows me to release any undesired thoughts. In those seconds, I feel transformed to ask the third step, which is mantra. Mantra serves as a powerful connection thread between using the breath, the mind, and the sound to call on a higher power. For some it may be a prayer, for others a song or a sutra. My mantra was taught to me as a child from the Bible, and I have never forgotten it: 'For with God nothing shall be impossible.' Luke 1:37. This helps me realize that there is something more powerful than this moment. There is a force greater than whatever problem that I am facing. Ultimately, there will be a resolution. Breathing, reflection, and mantra consistently match with what I was taught during the breath, water, and sound training and have worked for me throughout many different challenges in life.

Your mirror will be your friends, your lovers, your living space, your actions, and everything about your outside world. *Yoga is my mirror to facilitate change."*

Alanna Kaivalya speaks of a friend who introduced her to yoga as a tool to address something negative that was happening in her life. Once you see the life-changing effects of a regular practice, I know you will do the same for a friend of yours. What I found even more interesting in Alanna's story was that she understands that yoga, while introduced to her by her friend, really picked her. It's no coincidence that many of the teachers in this book shared similar stories of loving friends or family who gave them the great gift of this introduction. Some also call this friend cancer, depression, divorce, pain, or some other event that forever changed their life. Yoga picks you.

Alanna Kaivalya

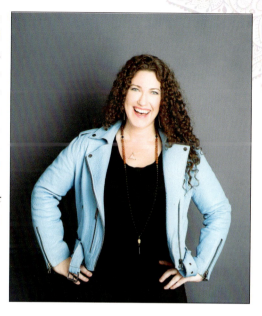

"I had just been diagnosed with Hashimoto's thyroiditis, and my friend said that yoga would really help. I was extremely skeptical because, at the time, I was studying physics in college and had little understanding of Eastern thought and kept passing it off as too *woo woo* for me! He finally got me to go to a class, and, well, that was it. I was hooked immediately.

Yoga picked me. Yoga is a *way of life*. It's snuck into every pore and cell to recraft the system from the inside out. There's no way to see life any other way than through the lens of yoga at this point. **You are whole, complete, and perfect. The end.**

Everything that occurs in life presents itself as an opportunity for us to practice. Any time we encounter resistance in ourselves or in life, we can see where the ties of karma still bind us, and this is essential information for the yogi.

Keep going. Yoga is an infinite wellspring of wisdom and transformation, but it takes time and consistency. You'll start to notice small changes, but as you continue, after a matter of years, you'll look back and realize that you've become a more shining example of yourself. You'll be comfortable with who you are, more at ease with your body and mind, and deeply connected to your spirit. This is the practice of a lifetime. So dedicate yourself to it . . . you'll be thanking yourself for a long time that you did!"

Yoga will help reduce struggle and suffering. Life stressors are a lot like waves. They can loll and lap at you, or they can knock you down in a second. Stephanie Troy understands just how yoga can help you navigate each surge and, perhaps more important, teach you about life.

Stephanie Troy

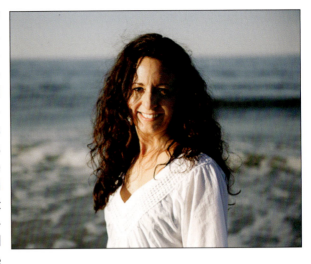

"I like to think of my current self as being a Type A person in recovery. Back then, I was unaware that recovery was needed. I practiced yoga like I did everything else: fast and heated. Despite the fact that it was at full speed, my practice was slowly beginning to bring me gifts that I didn't realize would be there. I began to notice that I felt calmer over time. The practice made me less wiry and more stable. I came for the workout and stayed as I became more connected spiritually as the hard edges began to soften.

Yoga has taught me that I desperately needed a practice to soften those rough edges. You don't know what you don't know. Back when I began, I had no idea that I was in need of healing.

Yoga has taught me a lot about life. Mostly, that life's stressors are generally like the waves in the ocean: they come and they go. Life is a lot less turbulent when I am practicing yoga and meditating. It doesn't mean that stress doesn't occur, because it most definitely does, but when I am practicing more regularly, I am able to handle it with more ease and grace. I have also come to appreciate life's difficulties as lessons rather than obstacles. I find peace within the teachings of the Buddha and use the philosophy in my life regularly.

Yoga is a practice that will help you reduce internal struggle and suffering. The quantity of stress people are under these days is overwhelming. If we practice yoga in the same way that we do everything else in our lives, then we have no place to heal. If you use your yoga practice to reduce the struggle internally, it has the capacity to heal your relationship with yourself, and therefore heal your relationships with others. Yoga helps me stay rooted within the storm of life.

Our society encourages us to neither feel nor deal. This is encouraged until people develop an addiction, and then they are demonized as disgusting and out of control. Meanwhile, most people are medicating away their emotions to varying degrees. Quick fixes only work for the moment, and then we are left with our unhappiness all over again.

Happiness does not always show up first. Quite often, my sadness or stuck fears show up for clearing. But, by linking movement with breath and flowing to beautiful music, I am able to detach from my mind and feel those emotions safely. The first time I cried on my mat was horrifying, as I was not someone who felt comfortable being vulnerable. I now cherish those moments when I can release through my practice. It is that release that allows for true happiness and joy to arise."

Yoga is empowering and can positively impact the spiritual, physical, and emotional aspects of your life. If you can breathe, you can do yoga. Among other truths, Kelly Larson speaks to meditation as the very core of how yoga manifests itself in our lives.

Kelly Larson

"When I first found the yoga that spoke to me, I was afraid of my body. I thought I was kind of weak, and I was intimidated by all the sequences and not knowing what the postures were. When I entered the deep, strong, slow practice community that is now at the center of my heart, I was still intimidated, but my world was rocked. I discovered a strength that I didn't know existed. I discovered the unrelenting life force that moves our bodies, despite all the fears that may try to get in the way. I found a new kind of freedom. And it changed my world in all the right ways.

Yoga will teach you to face your fears (the sensible ones—no hanging out with tigers) and take a deep breath into them. You'll notice how it makes you feel, and you grow. You will learn something about the boundaries that you have put on yourself. Yoga never stops teaching me. Yoga teaches about Life, and Life teaches about yoga. When you take a deep dive into practice on all fronts of your life, everything expands and becomes richer.

I have learned to breathe and *feel* when I am hitting an edge. What I discover is that, if I let down my fear and really breathe and feel what is happening in my body, generally the depth of fear transforms into a total bliss of sensation. So when I find myself in the midst of something nearly intolerable, I breathe. Deeply. I feel and land all the way into my heart's sensations until I can feel what is underneath them. Usually it is care, and it is love. Whatever challenges me is triggering something deep in my heart, and underneath all

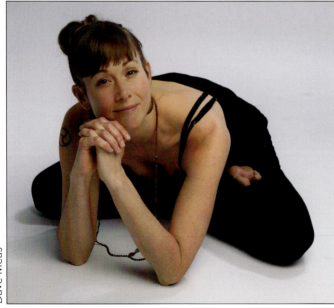

Dave Meas

of it is the part that cares and loves, and when I can notice that and breathe into the rest of the sensation (whether it is grief, frustration, anxiety, fear, etc.), then I allow the most challenging parts to blossom as they must and then ease away with my exhales. The trick of overcoming almost any difficult sensation is to let go of resisting it. Once you feel it, it has room to move. If you keep pushing it away, well. . . . That which resists persists. Yoga gives you the courage, the skills, and the capacity to overcome.

Yoga happens on the mat, but also outside in deeply natural places, on the sidewalks of overcrowded cities, and everywhere in between. And real yoga can rock you right into the reality around you. It's easy to be peaceful in a cave or a monastery, but it's not so easy to see pain and disrespect and the hard light of the sun shining on the underbellies of humanity, and still be at peace. But when you can let go into love anyway, then you have learned something about the beauty that underlies life, and you can be a bit readier for a journey into, and then beyond, your body. In fact, the biggest gift I have received from yoga is my capacity to relate to others.

My wish for you and everyone is to remember what an utter miracle it is to be flying through space on this tiny, gorgeous planet while we literally spin around a big bold star. And we are, quite literally, made of stardust. How does that happen? If you have lost your sense of awe today, consider going somewhere to gaze at some clear skies for a while and let your mind wander and wonder about where the blue turns to black, the shapes of the clouds and the stories of those shining stars. Because we are small, and our hearts and lives are big, and life is that f'ing good.

I will keep trying to live this miracle in a way that is fun, balanced, utterly beautiful, and respectful with every step I take, and I won't always succeed, beautiful, vulnerable human that I am. But if we all try, something very good will certainly happen."

Accept that life is unfolding for us just as it should, aligning with a greater purpose. A purpose that underscores that all living things need to thrive and expand to grow. I believe that Coby Kozlowski shares this same ideal in how she approaches life.

Coby Kozlowski

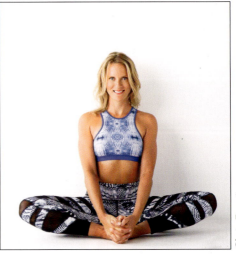

Chris Fanning

"Yoga has taught me about how to skillfully engage with life, how to 'trust' life (and point out when I am not trusting life), how to live on purpose, the art and power of true listening, and, really, how to walk a path of intimacy with life.

Yoga has taught me about possibility and potential, and that we are all being called to this potential. Yoga reminds me that we now have the chance to create a world of cooperation, collaboration, and celebration for those who are willing to show up to life. That the nature of the Universe is to thrive and expand, and right now in this moment, we all are being given an opportunity to shift and to step into a new current. To be part of this developmental process, we need to embrace and employ the tremendous intelligence of nature. While transformation may seem overwhelming at first, it really comes down to one small action step: a one-degree shift of change. In other words, you don't have to change everything to make a difference. What is the one-degree shift you could make right now? What small change could you make for the sake of setting a new course and ending up in an alternate place? Now, expand this vision even wider. If we all committed to one degree of transformation, what would happen? What could we create together? One thing's for sure: we would live in a different world.

Yoga has taught me that we have a chance to contribute to this one-degree shift, this vast evolutionary transformation, and shape a new life-affirming paradigm for skillful living. We have an opportunity to discover more joy and ease, and to celebrate the majesty of each moment—no matter what that moment brings. The world we can create—so close, but so far—is one I believe we all deeply desire. At times, our fear, quick judgments, and constant comparisons get in the way of celebrating our own and one another's diverse gifts and offerings. Yoga reminds me to ask myself and others, 'How can you celebrate what you bring, and what we are collectively creating? And how much more is possible when we align with our intention and trust the unseen forces of life, when we engage and participate?' One thing we find out is that we can't control everything in life, but we can take responsibility for how we react and respond to the various circumstances life throws our way.

Ultimately, life wants to thrive—it wants to find a way to make it. Nature teaches us that life wants to flourish. Think of a driveway with a crack in it—what do you usually see? Something growing! In the most impossible conditions, life still wants to live, to grow, to expand. Yoga invites us to align with this drive, with the intelligence of the universe. We all hold this flame inside us, and part of the practice of living our yoga is to engage with that inner light. You are the flame keeper, and it's your duty to keep your flame alive. It's a disservice when you walk away from your own inner radiance. Imagine what gets created collectively when we all say *yes* to our own little flame of life celebrating what is already in place, while still remaining open to growth and potential!

Yoga teaches me how to sit gracefully and with compassion—how to stay deeply connected and how to remain resourceful. I continuously ask myself this question: 'Why am I doing this?' And again and again, the answer relates to the fact that the meaning of my life is the meaning I choose to give it. For me, the point is about contributing, but staying true to this cause is not always easy, but definitely worthwhile.

Fire is a place of transformation, and yoga invites us into the flame. When I dedicate myself, I have an opportunity to morph and change through the heat. It is an opportunity to throw into the fire what I have been dragging along that's keeping me in the past."

You are a flame keeper, and it's your duty to keep your flame alive. Say *yes* to expanding into more, into your brightest light, your highest potential. The yogini in me, the yoga teacher, and the soul who cares about you promise you at this point in our journey together:

Yoga will help you cultivate the ability to live in the present moment. The understanding of living in the now is one of the most important things you will learn. Every moment? No, silly, it's called a practice for a reason. In its most simple form, yoga teaches you how to be awake. This is at the heart of the teachings.

If you can control your thoughts, you can control your life. Yoga will enhance your ability to still the agitations of your mind.

The practice of yoga is not about adding anything. It's about diminishing and perhaps removing obstacles, limiting thoughts, dis-ease, or behaviors that are a result of patterns that are holding you back from your authentic real self. Your best self. Your true self.

With consistent practice, the promises of strength, flexibility, and balance will be obtained. The bonus is a body that moves freely. The mind can attain a calm state. Stress is reduced. Situations that are challenging can be moved through with a healthy tool to rely on. The key is consistency in practicing the postures, breathing, and meditation. Living a life of joy, happiness, and your definition of unlimited potential is achievable.

The practice of focused attention brings many benefits: gratitude, a state of oneness with what is, and bliss. With contentment, happiness arises. Contentment is not a concept that is given: it's earned. You must have won and lost, lived fully, and been present for the good and the bad. The willingness to live in the present moment, fully, is a gift from yoga. Dwelling in the now, no matter what is happening outside of or around you, brings peace. This could very well be the secret to happiness: being content in the moment. Yoga will give you that.

My definition of enlightenment is being awake. You now are. There is no turning back. Healthy life reminders from your healthy life partner, your yoga practice:

- Stay engaged in your quest for authenticity, balance, and health. Make it a priority.

- Keep learning.

- Remain open, even to criticism. Seek to understand rather than to be understood.

- Be vulnerable.

- Embrace challenges. There is either a lesson or a gift attached.

- Speak your truth, but learn and practice active listening.

- Trust yourself. Ignore all the noise.

- Let stuff go. Apologize when you're wrong.

- Live from your heart in all you do.

- Bring compassion and love with you everywhere to everyone.

- Never give up hope.

Yoga taught me that there is a greater good conspiring on my behalf, something larger than I can define, that is light and love. I believe that I will someday be in conversation with my daughters. Living yoga, not just practicing yoga, gave me that wisdom and peace.

CHAPTER 11

You Arrive at Freedom

In the past, I bought into the idea that I could and *should* have it all (success, money, children, a husband, a full social life, a great body, *and* my own business). I used to believe and share, "You can have it all, but not all on the same day." What I'm not known for sharing is the fallout from striving to have it all and on the same day—for unconsciously chasing some perfect dream in a toxic nightmare of my own creation.

It's a tragedy that both my ex-husband and I were obsessed with having it all. Having both come from nothing, we were consumed by the idea of becoming wealthy. In striving to build businesses, we succeeded in deepening an unconscious metaphorical hole within each of us that we believed we could fill with wealth and power. A need for outward recognition of our value. There were no two greater egos, both jockeying for position; I lost the battle long, long ago. We may have presented ourselves as passionate and driven and determined, but for me, inside, it felt like crazy town.

A therapist told me that very few couples that jump social classes remain together. While I'm indeed proof of that statistic, I'm forever grateful that I've had the opportunity to start my life over, and I am also proud to call myself a PTSD survivor. It's been a huge blessing.

The Buddhist in me embraces the idea that suffering is part of life—it's our choices and actions thereafter that interest me. I'm not ashamed to admit that, when overcome by sadness and longing for my daughters, my *tool* of choice was alcohol. I've long since removed that *unhealthy tool* from my toolbox and put myself on a new path—a life of sobriety.

Is my life perfect? No. I still have my struggles. I've developed a creative sense of possibility that guides my days. *Action* is critical; I listen to my own wisdom, choose, and then I act. I still face fear daily. I still struggle to *feel* my bad days. I don't dwell there for fear I'll numb out again. I'm aware and I'm awake now.

Yoga is a healthy tool of self-inquiry that's helped me see that I deserve joy; we all do. The human experience may include suffering—but we are meant to dwell in joy. I may have been broken, but I'm not broken anymore.

As I've come to know myself in a much deeper and more profound way, I recognize that I need a lot of quiet time, and a lot of writing time, to force me to look at what's painful to see. I'm comfortable being a perfectly flawed person. I'm human.

Writing this book surfaced tremendous pain for me, especially around my daughters. It is my greatest, most constant struggle. While writing, I felt like I was moving through the stages of grief over and over again.

I'm more than a physical body; I am pure consciousness. We're all connected; it consoles me when I think of my daughters. I send them love daily. I sit, close my eyes, and *see* them before me. I pretend they're here. I smile; they smile back. That's as far as I've gotten. It's not much, but I believe. I believe that we will connect again someday. I have hope it will happen. I have a loving and supportive partner and friend who keeps telling me it will. Time will tell.

I hope and pray that my daughters' lives are filled with love and light, with friendships that are healthy and supportive, with partners who treat them as equals, with inspiring work that thrills them. As long as I believe they're functioning well in the world, I'm at peace. If it's true that *you get everything you use* before the age of six, then I feel happy with the love, guidance, and care I gave them. We had incredible days together. No one is a perfect parent, but I did a good job. I loved them and continue to love them.

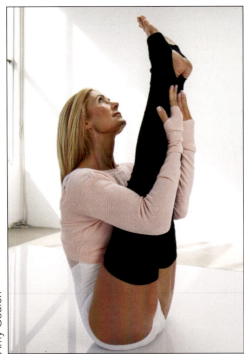
Amy Goalen

My greatest fear is that they'll seek out unhealthy life partners. The tragic reality is that's highly likely. As I type this, my whole body grows tense, because I know deep in my heart that I'm partly responsible for this. That's why I assigned myself the *hero role* of breaking free of the abuse that's been recycling through my family for generations. It took me years of therapy to unravel the mental and the emotional knots that kept me bound to the old familial

180 HEALING THE HEART, SOUL, AND BODY

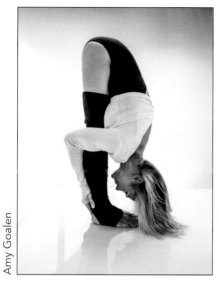
Amy Goalen

patterns and conditioning from a patriarchal society. If I can do it, so can they.

I still indulge in wild fantasies that my ex-husband will do the right thing and help me reconnect with my daughters. Surely, I wonder, someone must have told him they should speak to their mother. I can't even imagine what his response might be. That's not for me to wonder. I acknowledge the elements that make up his conditioned and patterned nature. I have the spaciousness to see both the conditions and context.

I know that the God of my understanding has a greater plan. I believe with all my heart that something good will come from all this suffering. I don't know what it might be, but I have faith. I trust the universe. I trust that love will conquer all.

My grief is present daily, which doesn't mean I can't move through my day with joy. It means I've done a lot of work to live with an enormous loss. I no longer need the pain to remind me of the happiness I felt with them. I keep a journal where I write to my daughters daily.

Michael often reminds me that I'm still a mother. One of the best Mother's Days I've had, since I inadvertently and unknowingly *left home*, was at a writer's workshop with the poet Mark Nepo at the Sophia Institute in South Carolina. While there, over Mother's Day weekend, I had the realization that no one—absolutely not one soul on the planet—can take from me my wonderful memories of being a mother. What a huge blessing. There are many days when I need to remind myself of that. I also have been given the great gift of being loved by and loving Michael's son, Matt. We're very close, and I'm incredibly grateful to have him in my life.

I still define myself as a mother, but I'm more than that. I'm also less. I try to remain humble and focus on helping others. I thrive when I expose someone to the benefits of yoga for the very first time—or welcome them back to the mat. I am at my best me when I try new things, when I fly high, when I dive deep, when I'm grounded and present in conversation with the one, great, true love of my life. When traveling, I am happiest. I flourish when I write, when I discuss yoga, writing, films and screenplays, and when I practice yoga—it's *the* most enduring and important and life-enhancing relationship I've ever had. These are all labels

YOU ARRIVE AT FREEDOM

of experiences—and *feelings*. I allow myself to *feel*. I'm not numb to life anymore. I'm awake.

My family of origin remains in my life, but I define what that looks like today. My father and I have had some amazing, revealing, authentic conversations. Do I still see glimpses of the abusive father from my past? You bet. Do I allow it to harm me? No way. I've learned that you can forgive a man yet still hold him accountable for what he did.

When I shared with my mother that I'd been raped as a teenager, never told a soul about it, and had suppressed the memory, she couldn't acknowledge what had happened. She couldn't understand why I was terrified she'd throw me out of the house if she knew. When I finally told her, she didn't ask who did it, or offer any comfort. Our conversation confirmed what I knew at fifteen: my mother was then and still is not there for me emotionally. She lacks the emotional intelligence to face what I've been through.

As I witnessed her squander her precious opportunity for awakening, I was moved to compassion for her. She did the best that she could with the tools she had. I know she loves me, and wanted me, very much. I love that she calls me at the exact time of my birth each year on my birthday. I love my mother.

Our lives are constantly bombarded with stimuli from which we react. When faced with life challenges, people often react based on the label they have assigned themselves. Maybe they call a friend in hopes they have the way forward, cling to the dogma of an organization for an answer, listen to the voices of their family of origin, reach for a drink, drug, or other method to escape making a choice, or have someone make the choice for them. Then there are some who simply speed through life, trying different things to help them make choices but never quite find something that works.

What I've learned is that in between whatever life throws at us, and how we react, is our choice. It's the one thing no one can ever take away from you. Recognizing that is not always easy. It requires you to be self-aware, accountable, independent, present, and have self-love. But when you do recognize that you own your choices, you grow.

I've recognized later in life that living a life of yoga provides me with a lens that enables me to make the healthiest of choices. Prior to my life transition, I didn't know it was healthy to put myself first—I had no self-love. Society taught me that loving others more than myself was the correct choice. My lens, before my crash, was through what society taught me, the voices of my parents, the needs of others, the needs of wanting to be a *good mother*, the demands of a career, etc. The lens was not from inside me, but outside of myself.

Self-awareness taught me to trust my own innate wisdom, to love myself, flaws and all, and to operate from a place of kindness and compassion. The lens through which I now make life choices is the self.

I could just tell you to go practice yoga, but I gathered these yogis who, through their own journeys, have all come to the same conclusion: that this system works. Anyone can do it. It's free. No one owns it. It's a system of living that will help you navigate all the parts of your journey of life. No matter what life throws at you, yoga teaches you how to make the healthiest life choices.

I've gathered them together so you don't have to crash. No matter how hard I tried to spare myself the crash, I'm grateful for the human journey. It would be easy to say I wish I had known the consequences of striving to have it all, but continuing to choose to look back is another form of trying to escape the present. I've studied my past enough. I no longer say *I wish I had*, *I should have*, *If only I could*. . . . I choose to let it all go. I made the choice to live in the now. When we accept the gift of being in the now, it leads us back to our authentic selves, only wiser, awake, grounded, and vibrantly engaged with our present self. In the present moment, there is peace and joy.

I've grown to love my unique, divine new voice. I've grown to love my body. I've deepened my connection to other people. I don't hide behind any self-imposed label of *good* or *bad*. Nonattachment has become a way of life for me. I gather spiritual wisdom from other writers, poets, philosophers, consciousness-raising leaders, and, increasingly, from my own intuition. I've learned to listen to and act on my own inner voice. I'm manifesting a life beyond my expectations.

I'm dwelling in the divine bliss of knowing I am valuable. I love myself in a way I never could have before. I've had the great opportunity to become the person I should have been from the beginning. I like myself, just as I am. I'm comfortable in my skin. *I know who I am.*

SPIRITUAL WARRIOR WISDOM

Looking back, one of the things I identified was that I had not cultivated a group of working mothers as friends. Women with whom I could intimately share the complexities, and joys, of balancing motherhood with a career.

I have since found, and become friends with, peers who are mothers and writers balancing family and career well. Erica Rodefer Winters is that kind of friend, speaking her truth and living from a place of confident authenticity. You may have to search, but healthy friendships are some of the most life-enhancing relationships you can cultivate.

Erica Rodefer Winters

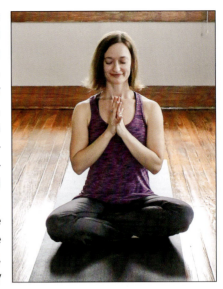

"I'm learning to embrace what Elizabeth Gilbert calls the 'beautiful mess' that is life and just be so filled with gratitude that I've been given the opportunity to experience it all. That's what yoga has given me. It certainly hasn't given me a perfect body, a perfect diet, or perfect relationships, but it has given me a little bit more appreciation for my many imperfections. I've learned not to take myself so seriously, or get too attached to an idea of who I think I am (or should be). It's always changing.

The other big lesson I'm learning is to love myself as I am in any moment—including those moments when I'm not who I'd like to be. First, I'm learning to accept and love myself on my mat, when my body doesn't quite take the shape of the pose I'm practicing. That has helped me to be compassionate and loving toward myself when I fall short in other areas of life.

Yoga is so often portrayed as this secret cure to everything that ails you—this mystical, magical practice that can help you become this flawless (both physically and mentally) version of yourself, which probably isn't even possible.

Do I believe yoga can help you to be a better person? Can it help you heal? Yes, of course! But it won't make your life perfect, which is the story you see if you follow many of the popular yoga teachers on social media. (The problem with social media, of course, even outside of the yoga community, is that people only post their happy moments and memories, giving the illusion that their lives have no challenges or flaws.)

For me, yoga is a tool that helps me slough off all the excess stress, tension, anxiety, fear, and self-doubt that accumulates in my body and mind throughout the day, so I have a better chance of handling challenges with a clear mind and an open heart."

Returning to my mat, my practice, and my breath is a joy. Finding and cultivating moments to build on and use to grow are possible for you with yoga. Embracing friends, mentors, and teachers like Lauren Rudick, who is living the life of her dreams with authenticity and transparency, will give you the extra energy to continue to unfold this beautiful system of living.

Lauren Rudick

"Yoga has taught me that the pursuit of my dreams is a very possible endeavor with enough hard work and dedication. Yoga has taught me that there is magic everywhere, and also that people are just people. We are all connected and all the same. Through my practice on the mat, I'm surprised time and time again by my physical capabilities. Through meditation and mindful practice, I've released the burdens of so many old stories. I have processed so many life events on my mat. I have found a greater ability to love. I have learned that there is strength in vulnerability, and that authenticity and transparency are the best ways for me to live my life. I have learned to be kind and compassionate when I am stiff or tired and realize that everyone has a story. People's reactions are drawn from their experiences and past traumas, and I must be kind and compassionate toward them.

My greatest desire in life is to love and be loved. I am so fortunate to love my friends, family, and students as much as I do, as well as to be loved by them. It fills me with gratitude and joy. But I would really like to meet someone to share my life with, spiritually, romantically, physically, and internationally. I'm ready to build a home with someone. My greatest fear in life is that it might not happen. Yoga continues to teach me how to release the burdens of fear.

Yoga helps remind me that impermanence is the only constant, and that even tough situations will pass. It also reminds me that I am strong enough to overcome anything, because life never throws at us what we cannot handle. When I am challenged in life, I meditate on a mantra I set for the day to help me work through and move on from whatever faces me. Yoga has helped me become fearless and strong, physically, emotionally, and professionally."

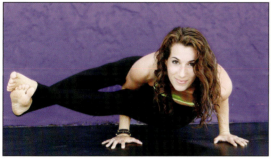

Dee Stecco

Living from a place that is connected to something bigger than ourselves is possible through the infinite wisdom of our soul: our connection to our own innate wisdom. One of my teachers during teacher training, Jenn Chiarelli, uses yoga to plug back into this ever-engaging spiritual connection. As she moves through motherhood, work, and family, I see her sharing from a place of creativity, knowledge, and embodied love.

YOU ARRIVE AT FREEDOM   185

Jenn Chiarelli

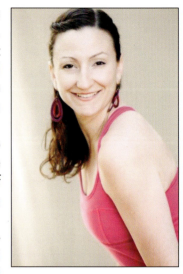

"Yoga taught me that there is so much more to me than just the physical and the mental/emotional. There is an energy that is available when you get very still. It is a powerful force that guides my life. I carry it into my meditation, and then naturally into my life. This energy has saved me from my own fears and doubts.

Yoga is not stretching. It is a beautiful and deep spiritual journey to get to know yourself. There are eight Limbs of Yoga, and the asanas are just 1/8 of the picture. The deeper practice is one of quieting the mind and going within.

When I am fearful and freak out, I know I am disconnected from myself (in the deepest sense). I know I need to get quiet and still, breathe, and meditate. Once I do, it is my way of plugging back into my source. I often tell my students that meditation is like plugging in your cell phone at night. If you do, in the morning it is charged up and ready to go. It is the same with meditation: if you sit every morning and connect to your source, you will be full and ready to give. If you don't, you're working on a low battery and have no juice or flow to connect deeply to life. Then you end up fearful, doubtful, unclear.

When we are connected, we have the answers, and if we don't, we will receive them when we are ready to understand them."

The peace, love, and energy I have received from surrounding myself with mothers like Jenn continues to remind me that we are all on this wild, wonderful ride together. Another mother, Tah Groen, agrees that we all have access to this energy. Like myself, Tah is an artist, yoga teacher, and mother. All of these labels are simply to identify us in our society. Tah is one of those people who lives from a place that has no label. It's an energy that I often label *kind* or *beautiful*. It simply means that the peace and wisdom and love that she shares when you connect with her in class is how she lives outside of a yoga studio. You can operate the same way off your mat as on your mat. It isn't something that you come and "do" for an hour and then leave there. Why not live that way? You don't step into the studio and leave that bubble of bliss you have created for yourself. With practice, you, too, will see you are a yogi. You always have been. It's just a new label.

Tah Groen

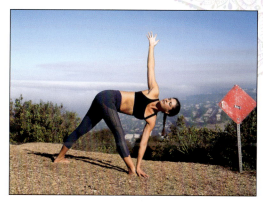

"As I surrender and allow life to be revealed to me, life gets better and better. The doubt and confusion lift to reveal clarity and wisdom. My energy, my frequency, my vibration become attuned to match my desires.

When I do, I feel good. I resonate love and appreciation. Living life fully awake comes down to that internal guidance and the ability to love. We are love, and we embody that high frequency. Its ability, the physical body, to hold the light of that energy grows exponentially as we clear out resistance in the body. Yoga and meditation can do this easily and quickly.

Yoga is supposed to feel good. It's not about trying or effort, it's about allowing the body to awaken. You are your own guru. It's about the journey, not the destination.

Yoga brings me back to clarity, wisdom, and knowing. I am able to let go of self-doubt. To connect to my true self the essence of who I am, that sweet space where I am now in love with life and all that it has to offer. A place of sharing who I really am: a confident, awake, and self-realized, teacher. Sharing what I know by being that example of sacred embodied energy, a frequency manifested through practicing yoga.

We all have access to the same source energy, and it just takes some focus and some training, and shifting of habits of thought, beliefs, and expectations.

Just by an hour of practice, you can shift your point of attraction to knowing this truth. I am Source energy, embodied here and now. And when I receive, I can give. This is supreme philanthropy. This is how man heals not only himself, but all that comes in contact with this energy."

We come into this world as a clean slate, ready to learn. The body of our teachings becomes our conscience, and unconscienced truth. Yoga gives you the capability to uncover that truth. As Sage Rountree teaches and shares, yoga gives clear insights and self-awareness, for you to be your best self.

YOU ARRIVE AT FREEDOM

Sage Rountree

"Yoga gives me constant opportunity to observe my habits, question them, and make different choices. It puts me in the moment, whether that moment is hard or soft.

I like to think yama and niyama cover intention, asana equals form, pranayama equals breath, and the final four limbs are all about focus.

I have a mantra, *form and breath*, that I come back to whenever I feel tired, confused, or disheartened. This reminds me to find mountain-pose alignment, or whatever the most efficient form is given what I'm doing, and to use a breath that serves what's happening in the moment. Combining those with intention and focus helps me be my best self."

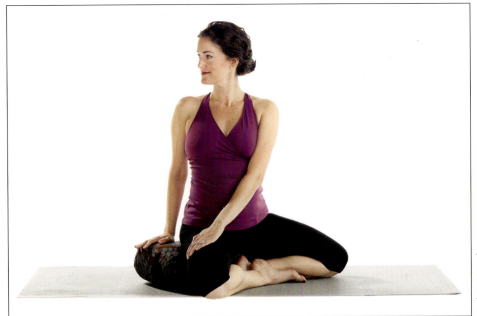

Seth K. Hughes

India Lee Benedetto knows, and shares, that yoga has a message that is far greater than our lives. As you come to embody the gifts of the practice, you tap into this universal message of our responsibility to our shared humanity.

India Lee Benedetto

"Yoga has taught me to first begin with myself. One of my favorite quotes said by Rumi captures this for me so well: 'Yesterday I was clever, so I wanted to change the world. Today I am wise, so I am changing myself.' There is always more to learn, and I have always been fiercely passionate and committed to continual growth and evolution. Yoga has helped me to begin to love my body and to practice self-care. Yoga has helped me to remember when I have forgotten. My life has been a process of remembering, forgetting, and remembering, again and again. Yoga has taught me about surrendering; to soften and let go. Yoga has taught me that I am strong enough to be vulnerable. Life doesn't require the amount of hard pushing effort I tend to approach it with. Yoga has shown me that to be truly free to do the work I've been put on this Earth to do, I must remain clear, and the only way to get clear is to get still.

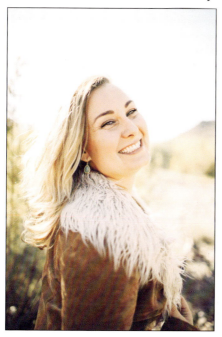

Yoga is a 5,000-year-old science. *Yoga has a message to share that is far greater than the separation of any man-made borders, world religions, or marketing ploys.* Yoga is about remembering we are all connected, and that when we unite, not only with one another but also with Mother Earth and all the plants and animals we share this earth with, then we are liberated completely. I want people to understand that it is not as difficult as we tend to make it. Yoga lives in the present moment. Yoga is about breath.

Life is challenging and unpredictable. Change is inevitable, and control is an illusion. Although our lives are in a constant state of flux, our breath can remain constant. My yoga practice has connected me to my breath in a way that is so conscious, it is like a metronome for my life. My breath is my guide. I have learned to practice Ishvara Pranidhana, or the act of surrendering to something greater than myself. I find great strength and peace in this action. The yoga community offers such support. To be surrounded by others committed to their own practice, who can hold space for you in a nonjudgmental way, is an absolutely invaluable gift."

Yoga is life. Life is yoga. You live yoga, so you live life. You don't simply want to exist. You want to thrive. You want to show up for yourself, as your best self. It's a warrior's journey. As a spiritual warrior, you have taken a huge step in a new journey. As Kia Miller tells us, yoga provides us with the tools to positively affect our life, our creativity, our purpose. This effective system can deliver profound results. I remain in awe of the beautiful love, wisdom, and all-encompassing work that Kia and the teachers in this book share. They love what they do because they have witnessed many transformations.

Kia Miller

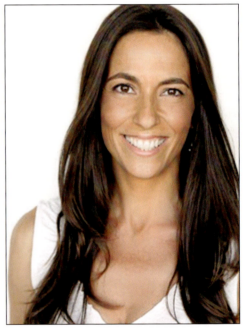

"Through the practice of yoga, I have learned how to positively relate to my body, my breath, and my mind. My body has become lighter, more flexible, and strong. My breath has become my refuge and like a trusted friend—I have learned how to work with the breath in order to change my energetic and mental states. I have learned how to use the breath to get myself to sleep or to wake up! I have learned techniques that enable my mind to be focused and calm. Having such a positive relationship with my body and my inner being ripples out into all my encounters with life.

When stressed, breathe deeply and investigate the source of stress or anxiety. When angry, channel the energy through your practice. It can be a great motivator. Once calm, investigate the source of anger and look at the situation from all sides. When sad and/or feeling down, activate the navel point and enliven your energy in order to swiftly move through whatever resistance has shown up. When confronted in a situation with another, ask yourself, 'Who has the more flexible spine?' Which means, can you bend a little and not need to be *right*!

In every challenging situation, the breath is right there. Just a few deep breaths can be pause enough to prevent yourself from reacting. Breathe consciously a little longer, and you will see different opportunities unfold that you may not have considered that can positively impact the situation. Yoga teaches us that all challenges are an opportunity for growth.

All of us are a product of what we think and believe. Through the practice of yoga, I have unraveled many of the outmoded beliefs that were negatively influencing my life and have changed a lot of my thinking patterns. It is in working with these inner levels that I have grown the most in my life. We each have the power to choose how to think, act, and respond to what life presents us in the moment. Our little microcosm of our yoga mat provides us with the tools to positively affect the macrocosm of our life, our creativity, our purpose. I am grateful every day for the philosophy, the practice, and the community that yoga provides."

Life is messy and complicated and wild and wondrous. This isn't the dress rehearsal, it's the play. This is your day, your moment. How are you existing in that? Are you really you, or a version you have been told you should be? Does the opinion of others mean more to you than your opinion of yourself? With raw and real fortitude, Nikki Myers is grateful for all of her life. She, like many of us, used yoga as a way to become whole and now uses her life experiences to inspire and help others. I need people like Nikki in my life. We all do.

YOU ARRIVE AT FREEDOM

Nikki Myers

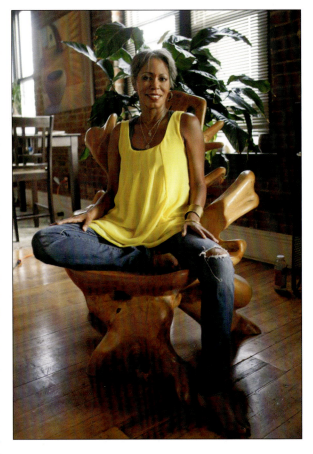

"I was introduced to yoga in the '70s and recognized there was something special and important about what I was practicing. However, men, sex, drugs, and other such things became more important to me, and I stopped practicing. In the early '90s, I developed sciatica, a condition that affects mobility, and a physician (to whom I am still deeply grateful) told me that while she was prescribing a drug to relieve my acute pain, she didn't believe that drugs were a good long-term solution. She recommended yoga, and that was the impetus to reignite my practice. And I've continued the practice from that day forward.

Asana, pranayama, chanting, meditation, and sangha (community) are all tools for deeper connection and integration of body, energy, intellect, behavior, and heart. When those begin to align, we experience a shift that reorients every dimension of our being toward a state of balance and wholeness. Often, even a single shift in perspective, muscular/skeletal alignment, energy expansion or contraction, behavior, or connection will realign everything, internally and often externally, as well. In that experience, we recognize that there really is no separation between mind and body, heaven and Earth, or me and you. From that place, giving to and receiving from the Universe and everyone in it becomes organic.

My work in the world today was born out of my personal experiences with addiction, relapse, and recovery. Through treatment for a substance addiction in 1987, I was introduced to the 12-Step program. It absolutely saved my life. And then, after eight years in recovery, on a business trip to Amsterdam, I relapsed. Gratefully, after much despair, I came back to 12-Step-based recovery.

It was during this period that I began a deep reimmersion in the study of yoga after stepping away from it many years prior. I stopped my 12-Step practices after a while and solely used yoga philosophy and practices as my support. Unfortunately (or fortunately, depending on the perspective), after another four years without a drink or drug, I relapsed again.

I am a recovering alcoholic, addict, the survivor of childhood and adult sexual trauma, codependent, survivor of domestic violence, a recovering compulsive debtor and spender, and a love addict. And today, because of the wisdom and practices of yoga, along with the tools of the 12-Step programs, I can say those things with as much gratitude and grace as I also say that I am a yoga and somatic therapist, an honors graduate holding an M.B.A, the founder of two successful business, the mother of one deceased and two living children, and the grandmother of five.

All of these experiences are a part of who I am. Today, I can truthfully say that I hold it all equally divine. I'm free from the toxic guilt and shame that once bound me, I am an integrated whole. Sharing that this kind of reintegration is possible for anyone struggling with what I've struggled with in the course of my lifetime is absolutely my dharma. I am very grateful."

I can't go back. Neither can you. Once you're aware, you have no excuse. But isn't that beautiful. When you see your truth, even if it's uncomfortable, there is a great beauty in that. When you cultivate acceptance through yoga, gratitude and calm become your constant state. We need all our emotions and use them to look, see, and grow. But Emotional Intelligence, the capability to recognize your own emotions and discern between different feelings, arises out of the practice. Many great teachers, like Giselle Mari, share that yoga teaches you to embrace "what is, and being in union with that (Emotional Intelligence) in a steady and joyful way, brings a peaceful life."

Giselle Mari

"Yoga (life) is a practice, not a perfection.

Yoga has taught me to listen more deeply to what is within and around me. I'm more attuned to subtleties and nuances as a result of my practice. Life is vibration—a big song, if you will—let go and surrender to it; you will be amazed at the gifts that land in your lap when you just stop trying so hard to make something happen and tune your instrument to the larger cosmic orchestra. It is all about being open to its magic.

Yoga is a reminder that my life is my ultimate practice. It is the practice of Abhyasa and Vairagya (practice and nonattachment). When we can consistently practice nonattachment toward people, experiences, and outcomes being a certain way—we can experience tremendous freedom and a lot less suffering. Don't try and make meaning of everything; increase your capacity to listen and feel who you are beyond your physical form. Sometimes life just *is*.

Yoga is our natural state beyond the ego self, which is effulgent, whole, and one with all that is. The practice of yoga asana is a way for us to connect on a vibrational, spiritual, energetic, physical, and psychological level to all that is. The practice provides us an opportunity to see how we are relating to our experience. Are we resisting or allowing? Is this a mutually beneficial experience, or is this about taking? What is our relationship to this form, whether we are moving into form in a class or standing face to face with another being?

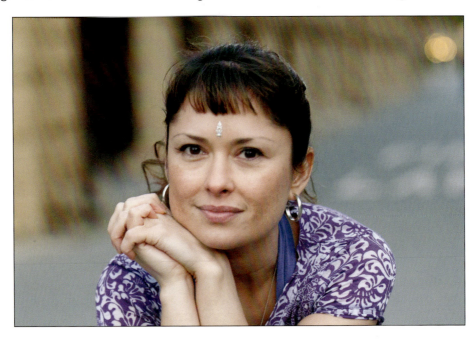

Yoga is a way of being that is practiced daily through thoughts, words, and actions. Yoga teaches us that we are all connected, not just human to human, but interconnected with all beings on this planet and every element that sustains us. It is our aim, as yogis and yoginis, to see all living beings as ourselves and ourselves as all other living beings, and to cause as little harm as possible. As my teacher often says, 'How we treat others determines how others treat us, how others treat us determines how we see ourselves, and how we see ourselves determines who we are.' Love is not limited to something you give, express, or do; it's who you are.

Yoga is about connecting to 'what is' and being in union with *that* in a steady and joyful way. Through continued practice, it deepens our ability to be one with where we are in the moment and also reveals where we are resisting yoga, or that connection. This resistance reveals itself clearly when we are in challenging situations.

This powerful practice trains up our mind and body so we develop a greater awareness of where blind spots are and our own self-made obstacle courses live. If we can develop witness consciousness, what is revealed is either our ineffectual habituated state of reacting, or when we are responding to our challenges with ease and equipoise.

Each day serves as a reminder that it's not the biggest steps we take, or the tallest mountains we climb; it's getting your shoes on and being willing to fearlessly start the walk on your path.

Practice makes possible, and when you taste possibilities, you've taken your first step into your unlimited potential."

Everything is possible. Anything and everything appears unattainable when you feel limited. I now dwell in limitless possibilities. I know who I am. I love myself, flaws and all. Knowing who we are at a soul level is possible, as Desiree Rumbaugh teaches. Facing a great challenge in her life, the death of her son, Desiree used yoga to heal. She reminds me that yoga teaches you to act from a unified place to create a reality full of joy. I continue to draw inspiration from teachers like Desiree who are using yoga to look at all aspects of aging in a very healthy way.

Desiree Rumbaugh

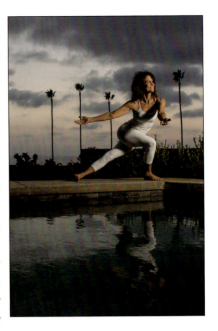

"Though we all experience suffering in life due to the human condition, it is within our power to lift ourselves up out of the misery by simply remembering, and then abiding in, the joy that comes from knowing who we are at a soul level.

I have learned to love my body, to look at my thoughts, words, and actions more objectively and with greater compassion. Now, I can see when I am causing my own suffering and make a choice to change the channel. From my study of all eight limbs of yoga, I now have the skills to work with my mind as well as with my body.

I am grateful every day for the support of my practice. I call it 'life support.' It has been with me and in me as I traversed through some very perilous water. Most notably, the loss of my son, who was murdered at the age of twenty. Like a phoenix rising, I have found a way back to joy. I am supported by a worldwide community of like-minded souls, and I am using yoga to navigate the aging process with as much grace as I can.

I use the practice of inquiry, or Svadhyaya, to question my thoughts. There can be no solution to our problems until we examine our thinking. We create our reality with our thoughts, so it is very beneficial to question them rather than believe them.

Yoga is simply the state of being unified in body, mind, and spirit. Even if your body is stiff or paralyzed, you can still learn these skills. It is a very simple, yet effective, way to upgrade your physical, emotional, and mental well-being. It can be adapted to any level of physical ability, and once you get the hang of it, it's free! No equipment necessary. You can practice unity of body, mind, and spirit right up until you die. You can practice however you like, and even if it is difficult, it will always make you feel better in the end."

Sarahjoy Marsh reminds me that, as a healthy life partner, yoga taught me to cherish myself, and my practice reminds me that self-love is an exercise, a priority. To love myself and others from that healthy place is my journey.

Sarahjoy Marsh

"In 1992, I was on a solo backpacking and adventuring journey around the country. I had recently graduated from my Master's program and found myself magnetically drawn to whatever might be next. I was, quite literally, free to explore both inner and outer horizons, the outer horizons being a practice field for the inner horizons. During this season of adventure, I found myself practicing yoga daily, and in expansively beautiful places: Canyon de Chelley, Grand Canyon, Yosemite Valley, and Orcas Island. As the months went by, fellow travelers asked about practicing yoga with me. Soon I was leading small circles of yoga classes. Far different, to the outside eye, from the yoga that I had led at the residential facility for our community with long-term mental illness, my inner experience of sharing yoga with others was nourishing to me and invited a sense of personal calm and quiet purpose I had not experienced often enough in my life.

Though the system is ancient, it is still profoundly relevant today. Yoga addresses human conditioning at every level, and though our ancestor yogis did not have to struggle with email and social media, they had to work skillfully with their minds and bodies to reinhabit ananda (consciousness, love, and grace) and to abide as that.

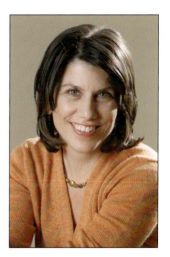

Cherish your vitality, nurture it, sustain it. It is the foundation from which we can give to others and to life. Open yourself to the experience of your humanity, our shared humanity; our lives are precious, fleeting, vulnerable, and require courageousness and community. The most indwelling truth in all of us is an innate radiance. It is too often overlooked, forgotten, or shunned. Yoga teaches us essential life skills, those that we need for the courageous and tender-hearted journey of living in love, for ourselves and others."

Once I realized I needed to share this great gift I had been given, I looked to teachers like Peter Guinosso, who showed me that the more space we make in our own hearts, the more we have to share with our community and the world.

Yoga is life, on and off the mat. We have an opportunity to leave a legacy of love. See this gift (yoga) you give yourself as a gift you give to the universe. When you are loving yourself, you are loving the world. If we can harness the collective energy of the world, we can shift our outlook from limited to limitless.

Peter Guinosso

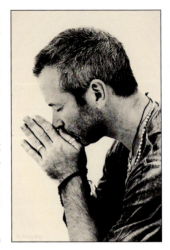

"As a yoga teacher, I have the great privilege of being one of the first voices that some students hear in their practice. The best part of my job is when yoga takes over and students find the authentic voice inside themselves. With practice and time, that voice takes the lead on the mat and off.

Growing up as a wrestler and serious athlete, I never imagined that I would find more joy and fulfillment in placing my hand on my heart and breathing deeply than I ever did in crossing a finish line or winning a match. Now I breathe up to my heart each day and feel a little more open with every breath that I take.

Yoga has taught me that we all have the capacity to heal ourselves and live in the present moment.

Yoga requires nothing but our own body and mind. The heart of yoga is a simple practice that can happen anywhere, at any time.

No matter what is going on in my life, I love knowing that yoga is there. Not just the yoga that takes place on the mat, but also the yoga that happens in the ordinary, everyday moments of my life.

The poses and shapes are definitely part of the foundation of the practice, but the asanas are really a metaphor for how we live our lives. How we do anything is how we do everything. Yoga can be the mirror we hold up to our life to help us cultivate peace and presence.

Yoga helps me slow down and look inside myself. In the beginning of my practice, the journey was about how I looked in the pose, and trying to get my body into the shapes. Now my practice is the doorway to listening to what my heart has to say. As I walk the path of my own healing, yoga has provided the toolkit: breath up to my heart, compassion for myself, and a community of likeminded souls who are also on a healing road.

Transformation occurs when we go inside. When we come onto our mats, we almost never know what we will find. It is comforting to know that all I have to do is show up with my tools: breath, compassion, a sense of play, and a willingness to try. The rest of the work is chipping away at the barriers holding me back.

The more space we make in our own hearts, the more we have to share with our community and with the world."

Acting from a place that is greater than ourselves is not only for others, it's for you. It's our job as teachers. What are we teaching our children? What are we teaching our communities? Sianna Sherman may have the answer. Sianna teaches that yoga is the path of direct self-realization. That by listening to the guidance within ourselves, we can operate from a place of love. It is possible for you. It is available. It is yoga.

Sianna Sherman

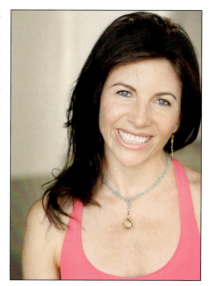

"Yoga continually teaches me that happiness is an inside job. When I get derailed with scattered energies of my own mind, I return to love as my central force and open my heart energy to the situation at hand. This way, I can hear the highest guidance from within myself and continue to evolve, grow, and transform in the midst of the outer circumstance.

Yoga is the path of direct self-realization, and allows each of us to expand our perspectives.

When I forget my center, I return with awareness to my breath, chant mantras, pray, meditate, and move in rhythm with my body. Yoga teaches me that love is my central force. There it all flows from here."

You are a yogi. You have the capacity to live a life beyond your wildest dreams. You are made of stardust, of light magic. I can feel the light and love when I am in direct relationship with my spiritual self, my highest self.

I am also in that energy when I am around people like Tymi Howard, who shares and embodies the wisdom that yoga can allow you to live in the world from a connection to a collective consciousness, a place of unconditional love, all the time.

Tymi Howard

"I started dabbling in yoga around eighteen years old, just as a means to stay in shape for dance, so it has matured and developed into so much more than just an activity that I do. My practice of over twenty years has been my constant means of connecting to God/Source through so many different phases, transitions, challenges, and seasons of womanhood and life. I know that the only thing we truly have control over is how we respond to the moment in any situation.

Yes, we must do the work and show up, but ultimately there comes a time when we must surrender to the Divine Order of things. The greatest of these letting-go moments is when we die, or when we experience our loved one, friend, student, or even a pet pass on. In each and every physical practice on our mat, we practice the natural cycle of life, death, and rebirth. There are no coincidences that this prepares us for all that is before us in our daily lives. There is no separation. When I witnessed the passing of both my mother and father, something that I have always said was my greatest fear, previously unable to comprehend how to handle losing my two best friends and greatest support system, I lived through both of these times with strength, grace, and peace. I know that my yoga practice had prepared me for this inevitable transition in life. I have a newfound freedom and strength that can only be experienced when

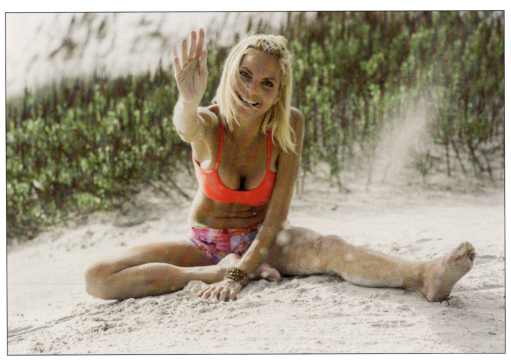

standing alone in my own power, backed by Source. In this connection, I feel and know that I am closer to my parents than ever before.

Yoga strengthens us where we need strengthening and softens us where we need to soften. It heightens our level of awareness and consciousness, so we become aware of when we fall out of alignment in our lives. We become aware of when we are reacting to things from a place of past conditioning, karma, or habit (as the witness) and in that moment of pause learn to cultivate and create new ways of thinking, speaking, and acting that keep us in alignment with our true nature and highest selves. We begin to respond from this Source connection and place of unconditional love all the time. All of life is yoga; there is no separation. I firmly believe that the way we do some things is the way we do everything; therefore, I am very aware of keeping my entire life on and off the mat in alignment with who I know I am, and the person I want to be in this world. Yoga provides all the 'tools' we need to bring us back into this alignment; we simply must show up, do the work, and be consistent. Yoga has taught me that change and growth are not comfortable, and that our challenges are our greatest teachers. Embrace the challenge and move toward that which we resist. Let go and release fear with the knowledge, trust, and faith that we have been given everything we need to do whatever it is we set our minds to do . . . and above all, do the loving thing."

At the time of my life shift, I felt so alone. There was a person out there I could have related to, but I didn't know her at the time. Now I do. Eleonora Rachel Zampatti shared with me that she felt her life was dependent on her abusers, and in that moment, I knew that there were others who could benefit from me revealing my truth. A great weight lifted off me, but at the same time, I felt a great sense of responsibility and joy. The weight of hiding from the world and from myself was gone.

Eleonora Rachel Zampatti

"I was abused, emotionally and physically.

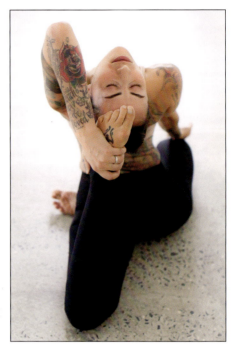

I was lost, and I suffered from depression, eating disorders, and panic attacks. I thought my life was dependent on my abusers, and I used to live in fear.

It took me a long time to recover and find the strength to smile again. It took a long time to simply desire to get out of bed in the morning. I was carrying an endless sadness inside, and I thought I could not live my life anymore.

I left my country and my family, and I was running away from a situation that I could not handle, hoping to find peace away from my abuser. When I arrived in the US, I was a lost soul with a broken heart. I struggled in silence, too ashamed not only to talk about my past, but also to think about it. I pretended it never happened. I never mentioned it to people, in an effort to forget. Above all else, I wanted to avoid judgment. I kept choosing partners who would hurt me, physically and mentally. I understand now that I did not think I deserved to be loved. I could not forgive myself for that. I was miserable and scared. I was trying to convince myself that I was okay. I was not.

I stayed in this darkness for a long time, until the day that I decided to take control over my life. I realized that the only way to break this cycle of pain was starting to love myself and take care of myself. It was, and still is, the hardest challenge of my life.

One day, after a terrible fight with my ex-partner, I found myself feeling helpless. I was in tears and drained. I remember watching a couple walking and holding each other's hands, and thinking that I was not good enough to experience that simple act of love.

While wandering around the upper west side of New York City, I saw a yoga studio. Feeling lost and depressed, I was convinced I could not survive another day in this world. I decided to just walk in that studio and take a class. I wanted to shut my mind for just a couple of hours and escape from the life where I felt trapped.

After that day, I started to feel the need to go back to that class, over and over again. Soon, the physical benefits turned into emotional relief. Through the movements of my body, I started to establish a relationship with myself, and I started to hear the voice of my soul. Eleonora, the warrior, allowed Eleonora, the vulnerable, to start talking. Soon, the two started to dance together. I started a deep conversation with myself. Tears started to flow, and I allowed them to just fall. I started my journey of forgivenes. Yoga became my happy place.

Yoga helped me connect to the present and let go of the pain of the past. I became so strong that I could not only stand on my arms, but I was able to walk away from all the sadness I was living in. I ended the abusive relationship I was trapped in without getting back into it, and more than everything, without feeling lost. I understood that yoga had changed me and helped me become stronger.

I wake up in the morning choosing to be kind, not only with others, but with myself. I am learning what it means to be loved, and I recognize that I deserve to be loved. Many times, I thought I could not make it, but I have. I changed my life. I did not let the pain of the past dictate my future. I choose love, even if love has broken my heart many times. I choose to believe in love, regardless, and it has worked. I now dance with my soul, with my breath, and with my vulnerability. I now embrace everything I am.

It is not necessary to be happy, healthy, strong, flexible, or in a good shape to approach yoga. If your heart is broken, if you are not in good shape, if you are overweight and you cannot touch your feet when you bend forward, and you just want to feel better, yoga can lead you to a different place, a better place. A place of ease, love, and stillness."

I always knew, when I started writing this book, that I would end with Eleonora's story. We all have a valuable story to tell. Knowing we may help someone, we have accomplished a lot. I will forever remain steadfast in a simple mission: to inspire others to use yoga to enhance their life.

Our time is so short, but my light is so bright. My days are so long because of yoga. George Bernard Shaw wrote, "I want to be thoroughly used up when I die." I want my legacy to be more than the abuse I once bought into. I want to be remembered as someone who taught others about yoga and living in the moment, for joy is there in the moment.

It's on my yoga mat that I learned how—by constantly returning to my breath, my heartbeat, at times placing my hand over my heart, forcing myself to *feel* it. It's not about the physical practice—it's about the love: love for myself, love for others, love for the gifts I've been given. Gratitude, acceptance, tolerance—these are gifts I've received from Buddhism, yoga, other writers, my friends, life.

Pain, both physical and emotional, has been my greatest teacher. Struggle, even while I was in it, has been my friend. Experience has taught me, *This, too, shall pass*. Any situation can be met by someone who's content in her skin, knows who she is, and loves herself. It's powerful. It's authentic. It's free.

I identified my dharma long ago, which is to share and inspire others to not only practice yoga, but live it. My hope, as you read my story and the amazing wisdom of the teachers who have guided and inspired me, is that you too will discover *all* that yoga has to offer.

Yoga has helped me create the most incredible life. I've been healed by yoga. I've been blessed by yoga. I've connected with others through yoga. I know and dwell in Divine grace because of yoga. I laugh and love and cry through yoga. Healthy, balanced, and positive things are in my life because of my relationship to yoga. I yearn for you to share in the wisdom and love. I trust and hope you will.

I am love in action.

I am light.

I am.

Acknowledgments

Thank you to the yoga teachers who changed my life. There have been many. I am blessed to have been allowed to be the Sherpa of some of their unique wisdom. This book would have not been possible without the inspiration and participation from the real, raw, vulnerable, and authentic voices that are here.

As I have come to understand, a book is a creative team effort. The words on the page are just the beginning. I would like to acknowledge and thank my family and friends who encouraged me to keep writing, even though I was terrified through most of the project. Karen Master needs special appreciation because her love and editing skills are exceptional. Kitty Knorr dived in and worked tirelessly on a tedious phase of the book. Claire Coghlan took my initial words and worked her magic. Claire's editing skills and insights were game-changing. A huge thank you to my editor in the UK, Laurel Kriegler, who cared passionately about keeping my voice, while teaching me so much about what the proper rules were.

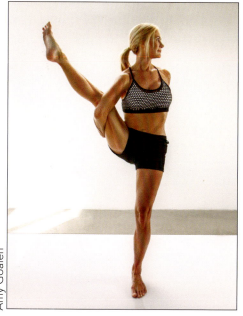

Amy Goalen

An enormous amount of gratitude goes to Tina Wainscott, my literary agent, who believed in me and the project and saw the big picture. Her love, support, encouragement, and professionalism is unmatched. Thank you to her, and all the people at The Seymour Agency, for imagining something greater than I could have ever thought possible. Equally important is my editor at Skyhorse, Leah Zarra, who helped me bring to life something I've dreamed of for a very long time. The day I walked into her office was a peak life experience. Her energy and enthusiasm are contagious, and I'm forever thankful for her confidence to bring this book to life. Thank you as well to all the hard-working people at Skyhorse who love books. Thank you for holding dear something I still yearn for and get great joy from, the feeling of a new hardback book in your hands.

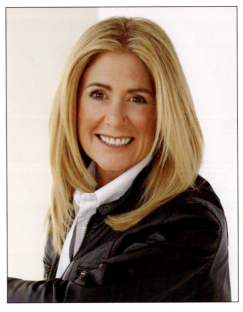

Amy Goalen

I would like to acknowledge and thank all of the strong, brave silence breakers who act for women everywhere who are silenced.

Thank you to my dear friend, Lewis Perkins, who is the only person who witnessed first-hand my life transformation: the messy, icky, awful days that morphed into endless moments of deep joy. His daily compassion, kindness, love, and encouragement allowed me to be myself in a time that I most needed one person on the planet who cared deeply for me, the real me. I am honored to be a witness to his life, and our spirits are forever joined.

Thank you to one of the most amazing men I know on the planet, Matt Orlowicz. Matt has seen me at my worst, and at my best. I have watched him grow from a teenager into a man. His old soul was always present, always loving, always caring, and I have grown to love him very deeply. He offered endless amounts of help on the technical side as well as the emotional side. He held my hand at the worst moments and celebrated with me at the best. I'm honored to share our lives.

Thank you to my life partner, Michael Orlowicz. Thank you for asking me very early in our relationship what no one else could. Thank you for your love and support on the many sleepless nights. Thank you for celebrating the wild, spectacular days, as well. Thank you for your capacity to organize and wrangle some sense out of my ability to put way too many thoughts in one sentence. Your vast world view, wisdom, insights, and laughter inspired me. This book simply would not have happened without you. I love that we collaborate on life and on other writing projects. Thank you for writing screenplays with me. You are the most exceptional writing partner, life partner, and man I have ever met. There is no one else as balanced and kind as you. I'm honored to be on this adventurous, passionate, profound, exceptional journey with you.

Contributors

Aadil Palkhivala is considered to be the teacher of teachers, since the world's top yoga instructors have studied, and continue to study, with him. Aadil has taught worldwide, traveling over three million miles since 1980! Aadil is the founder of the internationally renowned Alive and Shine Center™ in Bellevue, Washington, and The College of Purna Yoga™. He is the author of many teacher training manuals and *Fire of Love*, a book that provides life lessons from a yogic perspective. Aadil has degrees in law, physics, and mathematics and is a certified Shiatsu and Swedish bodywork therapist and a clinical hypnotherapist. He was a federally licensed naturopath for ten years, and an Ayurvedic health practitioner. Currently, Aadil travels internationally, speaking, educating, teaching workshops, and doing teacher trainings.

Adam Hocke has been practicing yoga since 1999 and has studied with prominent teachers including, most extensively, Jason Crandell. Adam leads yoga classes and workshops in studios and gyms across London, as well as yoga retreats internationally. Through a precise, accessible, and light-hearted approach, he teaches that we all are capable of using the body as a tool for enlightenment and healing. His unique, nondogmatic style is drawn from many spiritual and postural traditions, as are his experiences as a writer and researcher. Adam blogs and contributes regularly to *Om Yoga & Lifestyle* magazine.

Adri Kyser is an International Prana Vinyasa yoga teacher, Power Pilates instructor, and wellness coach who travels the globe leading master classes, teacher trainings, and retreats. Adri's mission is to help you awaken and reconnect with your Inner Beauty, while empowering you to live to your fullest potential. Her work has been featured in *Yoga Journal*, *Elephant Journal*, *YogaVibes*, *Origin* magazine, *Yoganonymous*, *Learn It Live*, and more.

Adriene Mishler is an actor and yoga teacher originally from Austin, Texas. She is cofounder of Find What Feels Good, a growing online library of yoga and yoga lifestyle tools to encourage you to be authentic, do your best, and find what feels good. She also leads "Yoga with Adriene," a happy and successful online yoga community that creates free creative content to inspire people of all shapes and sizes to connect to their body daily. Adriene approaches health and wellness with a playfulness and a sense of humor that encourages all personalities to the mat. Adriene takes her playful approach to yoga on the road, meeting new friends and connecting online relationships to real faces—always inviting you to build awareness, embrace individuality, and connect to something big.

Alanna Kaivalya is an author, mythologist, musician, and mystic. She is the founder of The Kaivalya Yoga Method and author of *Myths of the Asanas* and *Sacred Sound: Discovering the Myth and Meaning behind Mantra and Kirtan*. She holds a Master's degree in mythological studies with an emphasis in depth psychology and uses her extensive expertise in myth and symbolism to feed her knowledge of yoga, astrology, and tarot. Listed as *Yoga Journal*'s top 21 yoga teachers under 40, Alanna continues to lead retreats, workshops, and teacher trainings worldwide.

Ally Hamilton is the cofounder of YogisAnonymous.com, an online yoga studio with subscribers spanning the globe. She is a popular international yoga teacher and life coach whose passion is to empower everyone to live their best lives. Ally is the bestselling author of *Yoga's Healing Power: Looking Inward for Change, Growth, and Peace* and *Open Randomly: Fortune Cookies for the Soul*. Her work has also appeared in the *Huffington Post*, MindBodyGreen, *LA Yoga* magazine, and Belief.Net.

Amy and Michael Caldwell are the founders and owners of Yoga One, downtown San Diego's award-winning interdisciplinary yoga studio. After discovering the joys and benefits of yoga while traveling overseas, Michael and Amy were committed to sharing the experience once they returned home. Since opening Yoga One in May of 2002, the Caldwells are honored to have facilitated the well-being of thousands of individuals and continue to fulfill their dream of helping people live healthier and happier lives by offering a variety of yoga disciplines at their studio, as well as at offsite locations for various businesses and schools. Yoga One has been voted "Best Yoga" in San Diego for many years and has been featured on NBC, USAToday.com, Shape Magazine, *Fit Yoga*, the *San Diego Union-Tribune*, and many others. Amy, the studio's head instructor, has twice appeared on the cover of *Yoga Journal,* including their 30th anniversary edition.

Ananda Tinio teaches a vigorous, creative, lyrical, and intelligent Vinyasa Flow, informed by her study with teachers Vidya Jaqueline Heisel of Frog Lotus Yoga,

Jasmine Tarkeshi and Dana Flynn of Laughing Lotus Yoga Center, and Jill Miller of Yoga Tune Up®. She is equally inspired by the athleticism gleaned from childhood gymnastics, the infinite choreographic possibilities of dance, and poeticism crafted from her work as a writer and video artist. She has taught students of all levels in diverse locales. Ananda is in constant flux and embraces the notion of always cultivating the beginner's mind.

Anna Guest-Jelley is a writer, teacher, and lifelong champion for women's empowerment and body acceptance at CurvyYoga.com. Coeditor of *Yoga and Body Image: 25 Personal Stories about Beauty, Bravery & Loving Your Body* (Llewellyn), Anna has been featured online and in print at the *New York Times*, the *Washington Post, Times of India, Greatest, xoJane*, the *Daily Love, MariaShriver.com, US News & World Report, Southern Living, Vogue Italia, Yoga International, Teen Vogue, Well & Good, Yoga Journal* and more.

Annie Carpenter. Known as a teacher's teacher, Annie is the creator of SmartFLOW Yoga, an intelligent marriage of mindful movement with compassionate, wakeful alignment. Annie creates practices that are at once advanced and challenging, yet safe and playful. She has been practicing yoga since the '70s, performed and taught for the Martha Graham company in the '80s, and continues to be a dedicated student (geek!) of anatomy, evolutionary movement, meditation, and classical philosophy. She believes that yoga has a multitude of expressions and can truly transform and heal each of us, teaching us to embrace passionately all that life presents. Annie is the author of *RelaxDEEPLY*, a CD of restorative yoga, *Yoga for Total Back Care*, a DVD produced by *Yoga Journal*, and several SmartFLOW manuals. She contributes regularly to *Yoga Journal*. An influential teacher trainer since 2003, Annie leads public classes, 200/300-hour teacher trainings, and mentors young teachers in the San Francisco Bay Area, online at YogaGlo, and internationally.

Anton Mackey completed his 200-hour teacher training program in 2009 at At One Yoga in Scottsdale, Arizona. He teaches public classes, private one-on-one sessions, and workshops at multiple studios in the valley and is most passionate about teaching/creating Yoga For A Cause events (charity-based community classes). He also teaches 200-hour teacher training programs with a focus on yoga anatomy. Anton guest-teaches at studios and festivals throughout the nation (including Wanderlust) and leads yoga retreats around the globe.

Ashley "Puran" Aiken-Redon is an American native of the Outer Banks of North Carolina. An authentic island girl, she has called St. Barth home since 2005, where the majestic natural settings of this tiny slice of French-infused

CONTRIBUTORS   209

paradise have greatly inspired and deepened her practice of Kundalini Yoga. Her business, "This heart…KUNDALINI YOGA St Barth," was brought to life by an authentic passion for this exceptional school of yoga, a passion that she is inspired to share with others.

Ashley Turner is the creator of the annual MEDITATION 101 FREE Virtual Conference, seven bestselling Element yoga DVDs, and coauthor of *Aroma Yoga*. Known for her charisma, depth, and accessibility, she is a sought-after speaker, coach, and presenter. Practice yoga with her anytime at MyYogaOnline. She works with clients worldwide via Skype and leads transformative events to power points around the globe. Ashley lives by the ocean in Marina Del Rey, California, and in the mountains of Aspen, Colorado.

Beth Stuart started teaching vinyasa flow yoga after discovering the transformative power of the practice while attending college in New York City. She is known for her playful and creative sequencing, upbeat music, and contagious attitude. Beth sees yoga as a moving meditation and strives to help her students color outside the lines of their practice by inspiring them to be curious and open. Beth is based in Sun Valley, Idaho. Beth practices the yoga of mothering with her greatest teacher of all, her son, Jack.

Bethany Eanes is a yoga teacher, writer, and owner of The Yoga Harbor in Torrance, California. Life has taken her from a small town outside of Pittsburgh to the beaches of Los Angeles by way of St. Louis, where she met her favorite debate partner and turned him into her husband. She is as enthusiastic about breakfast burritos and sausage dogs as she is about parallel sentence structure and external shoulder rotation. Bethany is a storyteller at heart. You will find her yoga classes honest, down-to-earth, appropriately challenging, and full of story that moves you to contemplation.

Carol Horton, PhD, is the author of *Yoga Ph.D.: Integrating the Life of the Mind and the Wisdom of the Body* and coeditor of *21st Century Yoga: Culture, Politics, and Practice.* Currently, she is editing *Best Practices for Yoga for Veterans* and writing a book on the Encinitas "yoga in schools" case. She serves on the Board of the Yoga Service Council and teaches yoga at Chaturanga Holistic Fitness and the Gary Comer Youth Center in Chicago. An ex-political science professor, Carol holds a doctorate from the University of Chicago and is the author of *Race and the Making of American Liberalism.*

Cat McCarthy is a dedicated yoga practitioner since 1993 and innovative teacher since 2002. Cat holds teaching certifications in Anusara Yoga, Kripalu Yoga, and The Barnes Method Prenatal Yoga and has studied extensively within the philosophical tradition of Rajanaka Yoga. Cat's facilitation training in Conscious Communication via the NVC (Non-Violent Communication) method has taught her conflict resolution skills that she uses to bridge her yoga practices both on and off the mat. Mixing dynamic alignment and healing therapeutics with a playful approach, Cat's guidance is informative and entertaining. When not traversing the globe to teach yoga, this Emmy-nominated filmmaker directs and produces nonfiction projects.

Charu Rachlis has been teaching yoga in the Bay Area and around the world since 1997. Her teachings are influenced by the Iyengar and Asthanga schools. She has twenty-plus years of practicing Buddhism meditation and has been a student/teacher/mentor at Corelight—a nonprofit organization invested in raising consciousness in the world. She teaches in San Francisco and the Bay Area. She has taught at *Yoga Journal* for their staff for ten years and participated in the YJ conferences held in San Francisco. Charu has been studying and teaching nonduality for decades, mentoring people on their emotional processes and healing physical, emotional bodies.

Chris Loebsack, E-RYT 500, uses the power of yoga to create a space for students that cultivates trust, playfulness, and Divine connection with themselves and with community. Living by her mantra, "Clarity, Integrity, and Love," she draws upon her partner yoga practice to share the healing power of touch and safe intimacy. Chris has been featured in *Fitness Magazine*®, *Yoga Journal*, *Yoga Mentor*, *Good and Well*, *Local Flair Magazine*, and the *New York Times*. In addition to practicing yoga, she can be found rock-climbing, laughing with friends and family, or quietly meditating with her cats.

Christina Sell has been practicing asana since 1991 and teaching since 1998. Known for her passion, clarity, and creativity, Christina's teaching style is a dynamic and challenging blend of inspiration, humor, and hard work. Masterful at synthesis, Christina's ability to harvest and transmit the unique contributions of various yoga methods is unparalleled. Christina believes that yoga practice can help anyone access their inner wisdom and authentic spirituality and clarify their highest personal expression. The author of *Yoga From the Inside Out: Making Peace with Your Body through Yoga* and *My Body Is a Temple: Yoga as a Path to Wholeness*, Christina maintains an active teaching schedule, presenting seminars locally, nationally, and internationally. Christina is the founder and director of The San Marcos School of Yoga and Christina Sell Yoga Programs and Trainings.

CONTRIBUTORS

Christina Tipton was introduced to meditation in grade school and has been teaching health/physical education classes since she was a teenager. She practiced, managed, and taught in her mentor's power yoga studio for ten years before creating Imagine Yoga, a company that offers workshops that include a fusion of yoga and journaling. She also works as a director of admissions/outreach for Fusion Academy, a revolutionary private school for grades 6-12. She is a wife, mother, sister, aunt, and friend, and the only thing she knows for sure she learned from the Beatles: Love is all you need.

Cindy Lusk, PhD, has been a student of yoga for more than twenty-five years. She has studied and taught both Ashtanga and Anusara yogas. Her teaching reflects her love of tantric yoga philosophy and meditation, grounded in her many years of practice and study. Her students report that her teaching has transformed their experience of yoga and of their lives. Cindy currently teaches in Boulder, Colorado, and also offers online courses in yoga philosophy.

Claudine and Honza Lafond are the Sydney, Australia-based founders of YogaBeyond. Their love of movement, creativity, and each other has led them to creating the practice of ACROVINYASA™, which takes yoga from earth to air. Their collective experiences and combined career paths in yoga, health, and fitness have brought them together in a powerful way. Honza and Claudine's message of inspiration through playful practice has taken them to many places around the world as they continue to encourage others into a state of elevated consciousness.

Coby Kozlowski, a faculty member at Kripalu Center for Yoga & Health and Esalen Institute, has been featured on the cover of *Yoga Journal* and *Mantra Yoga + Health* and was named "one of the seven yoga teachers who have changed the practice of yoga." Known as a vibrant and relatable yoga and meditation educator, life coach trainer, speaker, and author, Coby is the creator of Quarter-Life Calling: Creating an Extraordinary Life in Your 20s and Karma Yoga Leadership Intensive: A One Degree Revolution and is a trainer for the Radiance Sutras Meditation Teacher Training.

Cristi Christensen is a former elite-level gymnast and platform diver who trained with the US Olympic diving team as a young adult. After an injury cut her Olympic dreams short, Cristi shifted her focus to helping others improve their level of fitness through personal training, Pilates, Core Fusion, and yoga. After earning her degree in kinesiology, Cristi studied extensively for more than ten years with world-renowned teachers including Saul David Raye, Shiva Rea, Seane Corn, Elisabeth Halfpapp, and Fred DeVito. From 2006 to 2014,

Cristi served as the director of the internationally renowned Exhale Center for Sacred Movement in Venice, California, where she continues to teach. When she isn't teaching, globe-trotting, leading workshops and retreats, and empowering others, you'll likely find Cristi dancing and doing back flips on Venice Beach.

Danell Dwaileebe is an E-RYT200 , RYT 500 certified yoga instructor. Currently continuing education in 200-hour Yoga Therapy. Danell teaches at the Hotel Del Coronado, Coronado Fitness Club, the beach, and at her own outdoor studio. Many years ago, dealing with a spinal injury followed closely by the birth of her two children, Danell needed something that would not only help strengthen her body, but also her spirit. To ward off any injury-related limitations, and to find her sanity in mothering two girls aged just thirteen months apart, she discovered yoga. Her discovery turned into a passion that led her to teaching yoga. Off the mat, Danell enjoys being outdoors, paddleboarding, fishing, and her great big family.

David Magone is the founder of PranaVayu Yoga. In addition to teaching weekly yoga classes in Boston, Massachusetts, David also films videos for the popular yoga website Gaiam.com and writes wellness articles for the *Huffington Post*.

David Robson is the director of the Ashtanga Yoga Centre of Toronto, where he leads one of the world's largest Mysore programs. David began a daily yoga practice in 1998 while at university studying comparative religion. After graduating, David made his first trip to Mysore, India, in 2002, where he initiated studies with his teacher, Sharath Jois. Since then, he has returned to Mysore annually to deepen and enrich his practice and teaching. In 2007, David was authorized to teach Ashtanga. David teaches workshops and retreats around the world and has also released an influential series of instructional videos.

Deborah Burkman has been teaching Vinyasa yoga since 2000. Her classes are influenced by Sri K. Pattabhi Jois and the Ashtanga system. Deborah teaches yoga in San Francisco and at her yoga retreats around the world.

Delamay Devi is a Senior Prana Vinyasa yoga teacher trainer, mentor, retreat facilitator, writer, and creatrix of Devi Designs. Delamay is a creative powerhouse and is well known internationally for her embodied offerings that are fueled by inspiration, deep soulful vibes, and infectious enthusiasm. She is honored to assist Shiva Rea for the past decade and is passionate about sharing movement as medicine and yoga philosophy in sync with the natural cycles of existence.

CONTRIBUTORS

Dena Samuels is assistant professor of women's & ethnic studies and director of the Matrix Center for the Advancement of Social Equity & Inclusion at the University of Colorado in Colorado Springs. She is also a yoga teacher serving in a donation-based studio and an addiction recovery center. Her book, *The Culturally Inclusive Educator: Preparing for a Multicultural World* (Columbia University's Teachers College Press), asks any educator teaching any subject (including yoga) to delve deeply to understand their hidden biases and to transform and heal themselves, one another, and the planet through self-reflection and mindfulness.

Desiree Rumbaugh is an internationally recognized yoga teacher from Southern California with an unquenchable enthusiasm for life, love, and healing. For Desiree, yoga has been a lifesaver emotionally as well as physically. With long-time studies in Iyengar and Anusara yoga, she brings thirty years of experience, experimentation, and creativity to her ever-evolving, outside-of-the-box style of teaching. Desiree travels the world full-time, sharing her compassion and her joy with others interested in the transformational power of yoga. She has produced a DVD series entitled Yoga to the Rescue and is a regular contributor to *Yoga Journal*, having also appeared on its cover. Desiree supports the Art of Yoga Project serving teenage girls in the juvenile justice system.

Dhanpal-Donna Quesada is certified to teach yoga in two different traditions. She feels blessed to be carrying forth the technology of Kundalini Yoga at L.A.'s Yoga West. Besides her background in the philosophy and science of yoga, Dhanpal has received formal training in the Zen Buddhist tradition. She brings the wisdom from her personal practices to her unconventional classes at Santa Monica College, teaching Eastern spiritual philosophy to large groups of curious young minds. Her writing can be found on *Spirit Voyage*, *Elephant Journal*, and her own blog, Leaves of Wisdom Falling. Her first book, *Buddha in the Classroom: Zen Wisdom to Inspire Teachers*, is widely available.

Sri Dharma Mittra, legendary yoga teacher, first encountered yoga as a teenager before meeting his Guru in 1964 and beginning his training in earnest. Sri Dharma founded one of the early independent schools of yoga in New York City in 1975 and has taught hundreds of thousands the world over in the years since. Sri Dharma is the model and creator of the "Master Yoga Chart of 908 Postures," the author of *ASANAS: 608 Yoga Poses*, and has released two DVDs to date: "Maha Sadhana" Levels I and II; and the *Yoga Journal* book, *Yoga*, was based on his famous Master Chart. Sri Dharma continues to disseminate the complete traditional science of yoga through daily classes, workshops, and his "Life of a

214   HEALING THE HEART, SOUL, AND BODY

Yogi" teacher trainings at the Dharma Yoga New York Center and around the world.

Donna Freeman is the founder of Kids Yoga Academy and Yoga In My School, two premier organizations that bring the benefits of yoga and mindfulness to children, teens, and professionals working with them. She has taught yoga and mindfulness skills to thousands of youth and teachers since 2004. She firmly believes that yoga can be practiced anywhere, by anyone, at any time. Her book, *Once Upon a Pose: A Guide to Yoga Adventure Stories for Children*, is a comprehensive guide to incorporating yoga into the classroom. She shares her life with her husband, four kids, and two dogs.

Doug Swenson began his study of yoga in 1963. He has had the fortune of studying with many great teachers including Dr. Ernest Wood, K. Pattabhi Jois, Ramanand Patel, and many others. Doug is a master yoga practitioner/teacher, philosopher, poet, and dedicated health advocate. He has incorporated influences from several different yoga systems, along with his passions for enhanced nutrition and cross training, to develop his unique approach. Doug has authored several books, including *Yoga Helps, The Diet that Loves You Most, Power Yoga for Dummies,* and *Mastering the Secrets of Yoga Flow*. Doug travels extensively, offering workshops, retreats, and teacher training courses around the world.

Drew Osborne is an energetic and fun-loving person. Growing up in the mountains of Utah, he was constantly surrounded by nature. When Drew was twelve years old, he moved with his family to Los Angeles, where he began to work as an actor. He has completed films and appeared on many television shows. After years of living in the fast-paced world of the entertainment industry, Drew quickly realized he needed a way to center himself. He unintentionally stumbled upon yoga. As he peeled away the layers and continued on the journey of yoga, he discovered an intense passion to share this gift with others. He completed teacher training and has since found immense joy in spreading the values of being a yogi. Drew believes yoga brought him back to his roots and introduced him to his true self. He found that fun-loving person again, in addition to new incredible friends and a healthy mind/body.

Dylan Werner is an international yoga teacher and advanced movement expert based out of Los Angeles, California. He teaches workshops all over the world.

Elena Brower has taught yoga and meditation since 1999 and is known internationally for her resonant, relevant voice. She cocreated *Art of Attention*, a beloved yoga workbook, now translated into five languages, along with a deck of visually profound Healing Cards to inspire daily practice. Devoted to meditation as our most healing habit, she's created potent online coursework and has produced a film called *On Meditation*, sharing intimate portraits of meditation from the vantage point of both teachers and practitioners. Practice yoga with Elena on Yogaglo.

Eleonora Zampatti is a native of Milan, Italy. She is an international body movement specialist, yoga teacher, author, fitness model, and founder of the Ode to the Moon project, a series of events that uses yoga, art, and music to bring about awareness of the topic of domestic violence and empower victims of abuse.

Erica Rodefer Winters is a freelance writer, editor, and yoga teacher who lives in Charleston, South Carolina, with her husband and two daughters. In addition to writing about health and wellness for a variety of publications (including her own blog, SpoiledYogi.com), she's also a contributing online editor for *Yoga Journal* magazine. When she's not busy writing and teaching, you can find her chasing her dog (and daughters) at parks, and in her own kitchen, experimenting with recipes that will trick her family into eating more vegetables.

Erika Burkhalter, MA yoga studies, MS neuropsychology, has been teaching yoga since 1999 and exploring its practices since childhood. Erika teaches Ananda Flow, a practice to "find your bliss" through vinyasa flow interwoven with mythology, mantra, meditation, and yogic philosophy to promote happiness, mental clarity, and a sense of interconnection between all things. Erika teaches for Loyola Marymount University's Yoga Philosophy Certificate Program, for Yoga Works, and for a variety of teacher training programs and festivals and writes a "Bliss Blog," ErikaBurkhalter.com. She feels fortunate to have been guided by such wonderful teachers as Dr. Christopher Chapple, Tim Miller, and many others.

Faith Hunter is the creator of Spiritually Fly™, a philosophy that celebrates every moment of life and uses yoga's tools of sound, breath, and movement in a fresh and modern way to encourage students to embrace their unique flow in life—on and off the mat. Her passionate and free-spirited teaching style is influenced by her study in Vinyasa, Ashtanga, and Kundalini. Faith owns Embrace Yoga DC, a training and yoga studio located in Adams Morgan—a multicultural nest of Washington, D.C. Faith has taught yoga at the great lawn, the Cherry Blossom Festival in Washington DC, and The White House Easter Egg Roll and is an esteemed faculty member of Yoga Nation on Tour, as well as Kripalu. She tours internationally, teaching yoga workshops, teacher trainings, and giving public appearances. Faith has graced the covers of *Yoga Journal*, *Om Yoga & Lifestyle*, *Origin* magazine, and *Sweat Equity*. She has also appeared in *Essence*, *Black Enterprise*, *Washington Post*, several D.C. publications, and numerous blogs.

Gary Chattem is known the world over as @ADevotedYogi. Gary espouses the view that anyone can be a A Devoted Yogi, indoors or outdoors, whether in a hot studio every day, relaxed in a zen-like state, or just one-asana-behind-a-closed-bathroom-door away from screaming kids, pets, and that damn TV. It is heart, spirit, and dedication to the practice that deepens the internal conversation.

Giselle Mari, E-RYT500, YACEP, and C-IAYT, is a global yoga teacher with spunk, spirit, grit, and depth. Her light-hearted but comprehensive teaching style weaves yogic philosophy, Sanskrit, anatomy, skillful hands-on assists, funky eclectic music, and an unabashed authenticity into her classes. She's graced the covers of *Yoga Journal* and *Yoga International* magazine, appearing in many of their articles. She's also featured in both Kathryn Budig's book *Women's Health: The Big Book of Yoga* and Linda Sparrowe's *Yoga at Home*. She's written for *Origin* magazine, *Mantra Yoga + Health* magazine, and *Yoga Journal* and is a teacher on YogaGlo.

Heather Sheree Titus is the owner and COO of Aumbase, Inc., producer of Sedona Yoga Festival, and director of MySedonaYoga.com; RYT. A passion for bringing authentic yoga to the global consciousness community across a variety of platforms drives her days. She is committed to building community and offering service in the worlds of yoga, arts, sustainability, and consciousness. She brings her project management skills to the table in service of this pursuit. Producing the annual Sedona Yoga Festival in beautiful Sedona, Arizona, with her husband and purposeful partner is her current dharma and passion!

Hemalayaa Behl provides tools to experience a balanced state of being, true self-acceptance, and a passion for life. Her work inspires and motivates many to live healthy and joyful lives. She is highly sought for individual yoga and health coaching, as well as major yoga event leadership globally.

Hope Zvara, "The Real Deal," is a yoga teacher, trainer, and fitness expert specializing in the true art of Yoga and Core Functional Fitness. She is committed to inspiring and educating students, teachers, and fitness professionals to practice authentic mind-body yoga and other holistic wellness practices.

India Lee Benedetto's personal yoga and meditation practice sustains everything else in her life. She believes that, in order for us to create shifts on a global scale toward peace and prosperity, we each need to begin with ourselves and allow that to ripple outward. India is a returned Peace Corps volunteer. She holds a B.I.S. degree from Arizona State University, an executive certificate in global negotiations from Thunderbird School of Global Management, and completed her studies of yoga therapy from the Southwest Institute of Healing Arts, where she now assists teaching in their Unity Yoga teacher training. India lives in Central Phoenix with her wickedly smart and kind husband and spiritual partner, Steve, and their rescue dogs.

Irene Pappas began practicing in 2012 and immediately knew she had found her path. She has studied in both Ashtanga and Rocket yoga, as she enjoys both a traditional as well as a spontaneous practice. Not only does she practice yoga, but she studies with hand balancers, circus performers, and contortionists to expand her own knowledge and explore the capabilities of her body. Irene's classes are a unique blend of strength and flexibility, always encouraging her students to find balance in their bodies and in their minds. Her classes are challenging in many ways but leave you feeling excited and alive, with new respect for the abilities of your body.

J. Brown is a yoga teacher, writer, and founder of Abhyasa Yoga Center in Brooklyn, New York. He is known for his pragmatic approach to teaching personal, breath-centered therapeutic yoga adapted to individual needs, including chronic or acute conditions. His writing has been featured in *Yoga Therapy Today*, the *International Journal of Yoga Therapy*, *Elephant Journal*, and *Yogadork*.

Jacoby Ballard is a white, working-class, queer transperson who has been teaching yoga for more than fifteen years. He is the cofounder of Third Root Community Health Center, a worker-owned cooperative holistic health center in Brooklyn. He is also the national program coordinator of Third Root Education Exchange, which conducts diversity trainings for yoga teachers around the country. Jacoby has worked with Off the Mat, Into the World, and the Yoga Service Council. He has received training by Kashi Atlanta, Kripalu, the Northeast School of Botanical Medicine, the Dinacharya School of Ayurveda, the Lineage Project, Off the Mat, Into the World, Yoga for 12-Step Recovery, Street Yoga, Insight Meditation Society, and the Challenging Male Supremacy Project. Currently, primary inquiries in Jacoby's healing justice work are around balancing self-care and community care, and holding both as sacred and imperative.

Janet Stone's studentship began at age seventeen under the meditation teachings of Prem Rawat. His reverence for simplicity and finding joy in the rise and fall of life live on in her practice and teaching today. In 1996, she traveled to India, her grandfather's birthplace, and became dedicated to the path of yoga. Janet blends the alchemy of her own practice with decades of studentship. She aspires not to teach, but to allow the practice to emanate from her, letting awareness blend with movement and breath. Based in Bali and San Francisco, she leads immersions, retreats, workshops, and more.

Jay Fields has taught yoga and the principles of Awareness-Based Self-Regulation to individuals and organizations for more than eighteen years. Her approach is gritty, relational, and intelligent. Jay received her BA from the College of William and Mary and her masters in integral transformational education from Prescott College. She is the author of the books *Teaching People, Not Poses* and *Home in Your Body* and is on the faculty for the Awakened Heart Embodied Mind Training in Santa Monica, California. Jay facilitates training and coaches all over the world.

Jen Vagios is a 500-hour ISHTA yoga teacher, holds a master's degree from Columbia in applied physiology & nutrition, gathers unicorns, and spreads joy. Her enthusiasm for life and well-being is contagious. As an expert in the field of health and wellness for over fifteen years, Jen nourishes her students' hearts, minds, and ears through her singing and teaching throughout Westchester County, New York. She has been playing musical instruments and singing her heart out ever since she can remember. Jen's unique "sound experience" includes singing bowls, harmonium, guitar, and her voice to serenade students into a state of pure bliss.

Jennica Mills earned her master's degree in social work in 2005, after which she began working as a trauma therapist in a sexual assault recovery program. Jennica is the founder of Brilliance Oneness Collective (BOC), a San Diego-based organization that works in partnership with community agencies and non-profits to bring affordable holistic healthy techniques to individuals, groups, and communities regardless of socioeconomic status, race, gender, sexual orientation, or culture. Through BOC, Jennica facilitates neurogenic yoga, TRE, and intuitive healing sessions with individuals and groups. She also facilitates workshops exploring the nervous system, the psoas muscle, and trauma in 200- and 300-hour yoga teacher trainings globally.

Jennifer Chiarelli is the founder of Anahata Soul and International Yoga and is a meditation teacher, mother, wife, former ballerina, and humble student of the world. Her mission is to serve.

CONTRIBUTORS

Jennifer Williams-Fields is passionate about writing, yoga, traveling, public speaking, and being a fabulous single momma to six super kids. Doing it all at one time, however, is her great struggle. She has been teaching yoga since 2005 and writing since she first picked up a crayon. Although her life is a sort of organized chaos, she loves every minute of the craziness and is grateful for all she's learned along the way. Her first book, *Creating a Joyful Life: The Lessons I Learned from Yoga and My Mom*, is available on Amazon. She has had her essays featured on Yahoo! and Dr. Oz The Good Life. In addition to her blog, she is a regular writer for *Elephant Journal* magazine, *YourTango*, and YogaUOnline.

Jill Miller is the cofounder of Tune Up Fitness Worldwide and creator of the corrective exercise formats Yoga Tune Up® and The Roll Model® Method. With more than twenty-seven years of study in anatomy and movement, she is a pioneer in forging relevant links between the worlds of fitness, yoga, massage, and pain management. Her signature classes and programs are taught at studios, clubs, rehab clinics, and medical facilities throughout the world. Known as the Teacher's Teacher, she has trained thousands of movement educators, clinicians, and manual therapists to incorporate her transformational approach in fitness and medical facility programs internationally. She is creator of the DVDs *Yoga Tune Up®* and *Yoga Link*. She is the best-selling author of *The Roll Model: A Step-by-Step Guide to Erase Pain, Improve Mobility, and Live Better in Your Body.*

Julie Smerdon is the founder and director of Shri Yoga. Julie has earned an Australia-wide reputation as a world-class yoga teacher and community builder. Passionate about empowering her students with her trademark warmth, humor, and enthusiasm, Julie presents the practice of yoga in a way that is holistic, relevant, and accessible to everyone. Julie leads teacher trainings, workshops, and retreats in Australia and abroad.

Justin Kaliszewski, author of *Outlaw Protocol: How to Live As an Outlaw Without Becoming a Criminal*, is a reformed meathead and former amateur cage fighter. He brings a lifetime of travel and a world's worth of experience in battling the ego to the mat. An avid student, artist, and treasure hunter, he infuses creativity and perseverance into his teachings, along with a distinct blend of humor and wisdom that redefines what it means to be an Outlaw and a yogi. He teaches Outlaw Yoga across the country and on the OUTLAW Yoga channel and is happy to call Denver home for now.

Karina Ayn Mirsky, MA, E-RYT, is the founder of Sangha Yoga, a faculty member of the Himalayan Institute, and a presence on YogaInternational.com. She is a Senior Certified Teacher of Rod Stryker's ParaYoga and holds a master's degree in East/West psychology. Karina leads seminars, trainings, and international retreats. She also has a telecoaching practice.

Karolina Krawczyk-Sharma, E-RYT200, RYT500, E-RYT., has been practicing yoga for more than thirteen years. In 2009, Karo started traveling to India, and that's how her life's revolution began. In Goa, she met her husband, Ajay, with whom she founded Bodhi Tree Yoga International School in 2010. In 2012, they decided to create a new independent project focused on health, yoga, and social work—in cooperation with "Loving Lap" N.G.O., they founded Trimurti Yoga. Karolina is a Type 1 diabetic; therefore, her main focus in practicing yoga is *health*.

Kate Connell is the private yoga teacher's best friend. Through her work with You & the Yoga Mat, she provides mentorship, trainings, and tools for yoga teachers interested in mastering the art of teaching individualized yoga sessions and the business behind a sustainable private teaching practice. She is the author of a book on the topic of (you guessed it!) private yoga, *The Art of Teaching Private Yoga: Teaching Technique and Business Know-How for the Private Yoga Teacher*.

Kate Kendall's approach to yoga is down-to-earth, lighthearted, and fun. Kate is the founder and director of Yoga at Flow Athletic. She regularly contributes to *Body+Soul* as their resident Yoga Guru, inspiring millions of Australians with the opportunity to experience yoga progressively and be adaptable to a contemporary lifestyle. Kate works with several well-known media personalities and athletes, and in her role as yoga director at Paddington's Flow Athletic, Kate has pioneered Broga. Kate's classes are regularly featured on MyYogaOnline and has been a headlining teacher at Wanderlust.

Kathryn Budig is an internationally celebrated yoga teacher and author known for her accessibility, humor, and ability to empower her students through her message, "aim true." With over a decade of experience in her field, she is the yoga contributor to *Women's Health* magazine, writes for *Yoga Journal*, and serves on the Yahoo! Health advisory board, in addition to contributing regular recipes. She is also the founder of her animal project, Poses for Paws. She is the creator of the Aim True Yoga DVD produced by Gaiam, author of *The Women's Health Big Book of Yoga*, and author of *Aim True*, published by William Morrow, an imprint of HarperCollins.

Kelly Larson, MA, PhDc, CYT, is passionate about delivering experiences that change people's lives. As the founder and managing director of the Center for

CONTRIBUTORS   221

Yoga Medicine, and founder of the Power Yin Yoga tradition, she is an acclaimed yoga and meditation teacher, speaker, and scholar. She has been featured internationally in leading magazines, and is known for bringing a fresh perspective to the topics of whole health, wellness, and personal transformation. She has been teaching yoga and meditation for more than fifteen years and travels the world to speak, teach workshops and lead retreats, and deliver premium private yoga sessions.

Kia Miller grew up in the Falkland Islands, riding horses over vast acres of wild land. Moving to England at fifteen, she soon joyfully discovered yoga and has been studying with world-renowned teachers in India, Europe, and the US ever since. A successful model and filmmaker, Kia has traveled all over the world, experiencing many different cultures and ways of life. She is passionate about living and breathing yoga and feels the teachings are a blessing for all. She is certified in the Ashtanga/Vinyasa Flow tradition, as well as Kundalini Yoga as taught by Yogi Bhajan. Kia is a devoted yogini and teacher who imparts her wonderful passion for life and well-being in her teaching. Her style pulls from multiple yogic disciplines and is both intuitive and steeped in the traditional aspects of yoga. Her classes focus on breath, alignment, and the interconnection between mind, body, and spirit, allowing students to work at their own pace in a safe and transformational environment. Kia views the science and spirituality of yoga as a path to exploring our inner selves and elevating our consciousness, while creating a counterbalance to the stresses of modern life. Kia's mission in life is to inspire, elevate, and educate as many people as possible, to encourage all to live to their fullest, most creative, and most joyful potential.

Kim Shand is a nationally renowned yoga expert and on-air personality who has helped tens of thousands of people "rethink yoga." Kim travels across America on a mission to inspire people to take control of their health, how they think, and how they age, through yoga. She motivates her students to find their power, their joy, and to be "All in. All the time." Due to a severe spinal birth defect, Kim began her yoga journey at the age of five as an Iyengar yogini. She later became certified in, and taught, Baptiste Power Yoga and Core Strength Vinyasa. Kim began developing the Rethink Yoga practice by fusing these styles with the holistic techniques of yoga therapy and the Rajanaka Tantra philosophies she continues to study.

Konstantin "Kosta" Miachin is the founder of the Vikasa Yoga style. He resides in Koh Samui most of the year, when he is not training or teaching in other countries. Kosta's passion for yoga blossomed in 2004, when he set out on his own journey of self-discovery. This journey has taken him to the far reaches of the world, from remote Himalayan ashrams to his initiation by a master monk in a sacred Sak-Yant ceremony in the North East of Thailand. He has undergone extensive training and is certified with five different schools—Yoga 23, Sivananda Yoga, MysoreAshtanga Vinyasa Yoga, Andiappan Yoga, and Universal Yoga—and maintains close ties to many other yoga schools around the world.

Kristin McGee is a yoga and Pilates instructor in New York City. She's also a mom to her son, Timothy, a contributing editor at *Health*, a brand ambassador for C9 by Target, and has appeared frequently on television, including the *Today Show*, *Good Morning America*, *Early Show*, CNN, and Fox News, among other programs. Whether working privately, watching her DVD, or working out in one of her classes, she helps you get in shape and have fun while doing it. Kristin aims to make her programs fun and accessible to all, beginner yogis included.

Laura Plumb is an international teacher of Yoga, Ayurveda, and Jyotish: time-tested and evidence-based pathways to healing, wholeness, and self-actualization. Dedicated to engaging the Spirit for Whole Being Wellness, and having worked for decades in the fields of health and human potential, Laura has studied the world over with some of the greatest luminaries of our time. Laura is the author of the bestselling book *Ayurvedic Cooking for Beginners* and is writer and host of the international TV series *VedaCleanse and Divine Yoga.*

Lauren Rudick's love of yoga has taken her around the world. She has studied, taught, and practiced yoga across six continents and in over two dozen countries. Lauren's appetite for yoga and travel are insatiable. She has been teaching and practicing yoga for over a decade and continues to train with world-class and inspiring teachers whenever she can. She has solid roots in traditional Hatha Yoga, Vinyasa, and Power Yoga, with continued education in Ashtanga, Yin, and Anusara.

Liz Terry, founder of Satya Flow Yoga, is an energetic Vinyasa and Yin Yoga Teacher (E-RYT500) who takes her classes beyond the image of what yoga is supposed to be and encourages her students to define yoga in their own way. She began teaching in 2009 and has been practicing yoga consistently since 2005. Yoga has taken Liz all over the world, landing currently in Dubai. She hosts retreats all over the world and is one of the Middle East's leading yoga teachers in bringing the world's top yoga teacher trainings to Dubai. Liz's teaching is dynamic, bringing techniques from all yoga styles into each class, empowering her students to take yoga beyond the mat and discover their true inner power.

CONTRIBUTORS

Lori Tindall is a yoga teacher, holistic nutritionist, and wellness & vitality coach. She is a human BEing, yogini, athlete, friend, foodie, health nut, lifelong learner, cosmic, and eternal. As she was born to a Native American astrologer mother and a Scotch/Irish cowboy father, this blending of duality is present in her life and teachings. Her athletic pursuits are bookended with chronic illness, and it is both inner strength and softness that best define her.

MacKenzie Miller is a certified personal trainer and yoga instructor. Her teaching combines a thorough understanding of alignment and anatomy with the joy of balance and movement. She engages deeply with her students in workshops worldwide and classes online. Her classes are thoughtfully sequenced, creating a safe space to have fun and explore, work hard, yet find softness and embrace vulnerability.

Margaret Burns Vap is a former city girl fashionista-turned-yoga entrepreneur and chaturanga cowgirl. As the boss mare of Big Sky Yoga and creator of Cowgirl Yoga™, she infuses her love of yoga, horses, and Montana into every retreat. She lives in the Montana mountains with her husband, daughter, an English Mastiff, and an equine herd. She shares her musings on life under the Big Sky, yoga, motherhood, and more on her Cowgirl Yoga blog. Margaret also leads yoga retreats internationally and is the founder of Cowgirls vs. Cancer, a non-profit that provides healing with horses and yoga to women with breast cancer.

Maria Santoferraro, joy spreader, E-RYT500 yoga teacher, storyteller, and always a practicing yoga student, lives near the beautiful shores of Lake Erie, Ohio. A former stressed-out corporate marketing executive, she is now living a balanced and blissful life, teaching beach yoga, leading international WOWYoga (Women of Wisdom) yoga retreats, and yoga teacher training programs, providing yoga and meditation videos and inspiration on her award-winning blog, Daily Downward Dog.

Mark Shveima entered the arena of yoga in tandem with martial arts at the tailend of a career as a heavy metal vocalist. From his beginning studies in Philadelphia, he moved to San Francisco. There, he spent six years diving deep into practice and study, guided by a succession of intelligent, gifted teachers in a variety of styles and his own daily study and practice. This led to his entry into an initiatory study of nondual Tantra Shaiva, Indian philosophy, and meditation with Paul Muller-Ortega. In 2008, he made a Hanuman leap to Kyoto, Japan, where he is the coowner and Yoga Director of studio BiNDU, nestled in the quiet back streets of a cultural center of Kyoto.

Mas Vidal is a yogi, mystic, practitioner of Ayurveda and founder/director of Dancing Shiva Yoga Ayurveda, an international nonprofit educational organization based in southern California. His vision for a better today is focused on social and personal transformation through a balanced lifestyle according to the natural laws taught in Ayurveda. His teachings propagate the importance of individuality, responsibility, and reflection through classical yoga to accentuate deep personal healing. He is a pioneer teacher and lecturer of yoga and Ayurveda and is recognized internationally for his work in propagating a unified approach to these sister sciences. His teachings are creative and dynamic expressions of various yoga systems that also embrace the wisdom of an Ayurvedic lifestyle. His teachings and main educational influence is of the lineage of Paramahansa Yogananda of the Self Realization Fellowship. Mas teaches the original Yoga and Ayurveda Lifestyle and Therapy Certification programs internationally, and as an Ayurvedic practitioner, he maintains an active clinical practice.

Meg Pearson is a nutritarian, passionate raw vegan chef and plant-based food educator, yoga teacher, Reiki practitioner, inspirational speaker, cookbook author, and eating disorder awareness advocate, with a personal mission to make the world a sweeter place, filled with love. Meg's yoga practice has been an integral part of her day-to-day life for a decade, and she holds over 200+ hours in vinyasa flow and YogaFit Canada certification. Meg currently resides in Costa Rica, where she leads raw food classes and retreats and offers private chef services and yoga sessions.

Melissa Smith is a Yoga Alliance ERYT® 500 in yoga therapeutics, yoga teacher trainer with Yogshakti and Holistic Yoga Teacher Training, Thai Yoga Massage, and AcroYoga® Level 2 Certified Teacher. A native Texan, Melissa currently lives in Kuala Lumpur, Malaysia, with her two sons and leads Love and Service Retreats in Southeast Asia and the United States.

Melody Moore, PhD, RYT, is a social entrepreneur, a licensed clinical psychologist, yoga teacher, author, and speaker. She is the founder of the Embody Love Movement Foundation, a nonprofit whose mission is to empower girls and women to celebrate their inner beauty, commit to kindness, and contribute to meaningful change in the world. Dr. Moore's work has been featured in the books *Yoga and Body Image* (eds. Klein and Guest-Jelly) and *Yoga and Eating Disorders: Ancient Healing for Modern Illness* (eds. Costin and Kelly), as well as *National Geographic* magazine, *Yoga Journal*, *Yoga International*, *Mantra*, *Elephant Journal*, and *Origin* magazine. She created the collegiate BodyImage3D program for Delta Delta Delta and is their subject matter expert on self-love and body acceptance. She is the National Eating Disorder Association's advice columnist, an advisor for World Muse, and a faculty member for Off the Mat, Into the World. In 2015, she was featured as one of ten "Game Changers" by the *Yoga Journal* and chosen as one of the 100 "Most Influential Global Leaders Empowering Women Worldwide" by EBW2020.

Michelle Jacobi, C-IAYT, E-RYT500, is the founder and director of the Centre de Yoga du Marais Paris, 2001 to present. She received her initial through advanced teacher's training from the Hatha Integral Yoga Institute founded by Sri Swami Satchidananda. "A peaceful life, a useful life" inspired her to become a yoga therapist. Michelle teaches and travels abroad, leading yoga retreats to beautiful locations and bringing the power of community to new corners of the world. Influenced by her Vipassana meditation practice, Michelle's Hatha classes accentuate fluidity and mindfulness in movement and breath.

Monette Chilson is the author of *Sophia Rising: Awakening Your Sacred Wisdom Through Yoga*. Published by Bright Sky Press in 2013, her debut book helps yoga enthusiasts meld the spirituality of the faith tradition with the sacred awareness cultivated through their yoga practice. She writes and speaks about faith, yoga, and the feminine face of God. She's written for *Yoga Journal*, *Integral Yoga* magazine, and *Elephant Journal*, among others. *Sophia Rising* was awarded the Illumination Book Award gold medal, as well as the Hoffer Small Press and First Horizon Awards. She lives in Houston with her husband and two children.

Nico Luce has been practicing and teaching yoga for over a decade and has trained in various lineages such as Power Vinyasa, Ashtanga, Anusara, Yin, and Pilates. He is also a devoted student of Eastern philosophy and spirituality. Nico's classes combine inspiring themes with a dynamic physical practice focused on refinement while cultivating presence in the moment. Nico lives in Lausanne, Switzerland, with his wife, Chloe, and their two children and travels internationally offering workshops, retreats, and teacher trainings. He also produces instructional yoga videos for GAIAM TV/MyYoga.

Nicolai Bachman has been teaching Sanskrit, chanting, yoga philosophy, and Ayurveda at venues across America since 1994. He holds an MA in Eastern philosophy, an MS in Nutrition, and is E-RYT500 certified. Nicolai has authored *108 Sanskrit Flash Cards*, *The Language of Ayurveda*, *The Language of Yoga*, and two books on the yoga sutras.

Nikki Myers, an accomplished teacher and practitioner, is a yoga therapist, somatic experiencing practitioner, certified addictions recovery specialist, and MBA. Reborn from her personal struggle with addiction, Nikki is the founder of Y12SR, The Yoga of 12-Step Recovery. Nikki's work has been featured in the *New York Times*, *Yoga Journal*, *Black Enterprise*, the *Huffington Post*, *Origin* magazine, *CBSnews online*, and more. She is honored to be a cofounder of the annual Yoga, Meditation, and Recovery conferences at Esalen Institute and Kripalu Center. In 2014, Nikki was honored as the recipient of the esteemed NUVO Cultural Visionary Award for her work with Y12SR.

Pete Guinosso is known for his joyful energy, skilled touch, and sense of humor, and he creates a spiritual, yet lighthearted, environment for his students to discover the deeper benefits of yoga. Pete's ability to compassionately guide students of all levels through a vigorous asana practice makes his classes, workshops, and teacher trainings among the most dynamic in the Bay Area and around the world.

Peter Sterios is an internationally recognized teacher based in San Luis Obispo, California. His video "Gravity & Grace" placed in *Yoga Journal*'s "top 15 yoga DVDs of all time" (2008). He founded Manduka Yoga Products (1997), writes for various publications (*Yoga Journal*, *Elephant Journal*, *Yoga* magazine (UK), *Fit Yoga*, and *LA Yoga*), and taught yoga at the White House for three years for Michelle Obama's antiobesity initiatives (2011–13).

Rama Jyoti Vernon, internationally acclaimed yoga instructor, peace mediator, and author, was one of America's first yoga teachers. An early student of B.K.S. Iyengar, she sponsored the migration of numerous masters from India to the US. Rama founded the California Yoga Teachers' Association, whose newsletter was the original *Yoga Journal*, and her teachings shaped the foundation of contemporary yoga. She has devoted much of her life to peace missions throughout the world. Her work is codified in the ultimate yoga practice book, *Yoga: The Practice of Myth and Sacred Geometry*, and in her yoga philosophy commentaries, *Patañjali's Yoga Sūtras*, and *Gateway to Enlightenment*.

Richard Miller, PhD. For over four decades, Dr. Richard Miller has dedicated his life to the prevention and alleviation of suffering, and to helping people awaken to their essential wholeness and well-being. Founding president of the Integrative Restoration Institute and cofounder of the International Association of Yoga Therapy, Dr. Miller is regarded as a leader in the field of meditation, yoga therapy, and mental health. A respected author, scholar, and speaker, Dr. Miller leads workshops, trainings, and retreats internationally.

Richard Rosen began his study of yoga in 1980 and trained for several years in the early 1980s at the BKS Iyengar Yoga Institute in San Francisco. In 1987, he cofounded the Piedmont Yoga Studio in Oakland, California. PYS, which existed for nearly twenty-eight years, closed its doors for the last time in January 2015. Richard, though, still teaches five of his seven weekly public classes at the old PYS building at 3966 Piedmont Ave., now occupied by You and the Mat. He is a contributing editor at *Yoga Journal* magazine and president of the board of the Yoga Dana Foundation, which supports Northern California teachers bringing yoga to underserved communities. Richard has written three books for Shambhala, *The Yoga of Breath: A Step-by-Step Guide to Pranayama (2002)*, *Pranayama: Beyond the Fundamentals (2006),* and *Original Yoga: Rediscovering Traditional Practices of Hatha Yoga (2012)*; he's also recorded a seven-disc set of instructional CDs for Shambhala titled *The Practice of Pranayama: An In-Depth Guide to the Yoga of Breath (2010)*. Richard lives in a cottage built in 1906 in beautiful Berkeley, California.

Rob Schware is the executive director of the Give Back Yoga Foundation, president of the Yoga Service Council, and Seva advisor to the Hanuman Festival. He is married to Alice Trembour. They have three children.

Robin Afinowich has a busy Tempe, Arizona-based private practice, where she serves as a psychological and spiritual guide and somatic practitioner; and teaches regular yoga and meditation classes at The Laughing Buddha. Her work is rooted in sixteen years of study dedicated to various schools of psychology, philosophy, restorative therapies, and holistic wellness.

Robin Martin's yoga journey began in 2000. Robin received her 200-hour Yoga Alliance certification through Tiffany Cruikshank Yoga. She has studied with Edward Clark, Baron Baptiste, and Richard Freeman and is also an avid AcroYoga practitioner. While her teaching focus is vinyasa yoga, she is constantly exploring different styles and growing and evolving her own practice. She believes yoga is accessible to anyone willing to take the first step on their own personal yoga journey.

Rolf Gates, author of the acclaimed books on yogic philosophy *Meditations from the Mat: Daily Reflections on the Path of Yoga* and *Meditations on Intention and Being: Daily Reflections on the Path of Yoga, Mindfulness, and Compassion,* is one of the leading voices of modern yoga. Rolf conducts Vinyasa Intensives and 200/500 teacher trainings throughout the US and abroad. A former social worker and US Airborne Ranger who has practiced meditation for the last twenty years, Rolf brings his eclectic background to his practice and his teachings. Rolf is the cofounder of the Yoga + Recovery Conference at Esalen Institute in Big Sur, California, and brought yoga and functional stretching to the US Department of Defense's Tri-County Summit on Sustainability. He is pleased to be working with the US Military on sustainable care for the troops and their families. Rolf also works weekly one-on-one with clients in his Yoga Life Coaching program. Rolf lives in Santa Cruz with his wife and two children. He has become an avid surfer and puts his yoga to work on his board, and as a husband and father.

Sage Rountree, PhD, E-RYT500, is an internationally recognized authority in yoga for athletes. Author of several books, including *The Athlete's Guide to Yoga*, *Racing Wisely*, and *Everyday Yoga*, she contributes to *Runner's World* and *Yoga Journal*. Sage's classes, training plans, videos, books, and articles make yoga and endurance exercise accessible to everyone. Her goal is to help people find the right balance between work and rest for peak performance in sports and in life. Sage teaches workshops internationally and online at YogaVibes and at Sage Yoga Teacher Training.

Sarahjoy Marsh, MA, E-RYT500, and vibrant, compassionate catalyst for transformation to those who suffer, is a pioneer of East/West integrated yoga therapy for addiction recovery. Her book, *Hunger, Hope & Healing: A Yoga Approach to Reclaiming Your Relationship with Your Body and Food*, outlines her comprehensive and effective methodology. Committed to supporting marginalized populations and using yoga for social justice, Sarahjoy founded Living Yoga and the DAYA Foundation.

Sari Leigh (a.k.a. Anacostia Yogi) is a blogger, yoga instructor, and health activist based in Washington, DC, with a special focus of yoga as means of healing from traumatic wounds. Sari offers an energetic Prana Flow approach as a way for those looking for a combination of spirituality and wellness. She trained with Gopi Kinnecutt, studied under Maya Breuer, and now teaches in Anacostia, Washington, DC.

Seane Corn is an internationally celebrated yoga teacher known for her impassioned activism, unique self-expression, and inspirational style of teaching that incorporates both the physical and mystical aspects of the practice of yoga. Since the beginning of her teaching career in 1994, Seane has appeared on over twenty magazine covers and was featured in over thirty magazine publications. Seane was a featured yoga contributor for Oprah.com's "Spirit" section and was

CONTRIBUTORS 229

seen on *The Today Show* with Matt Lauer. Seane has created four yoga DVDs and one audio CD produced by *Gaiam*, *Sounds True*, and *Yoga Journal* and has a DVD on the chakras and the mind/body connection. Seane created Off The Mat Into The World (OTM), an organization dedicated to bridging yoga and activism.

Sharon Gannon is a twenty-first-century Renaissance woman, an abolitionist, an animal rights and vegan activist, and a world-renowned yogini, writer, dancer, and musician. Sharon is perhaps best known as the cofounder, along with David Life, of the Jivamukti Yoga method—a path to enlightenment through compassion for all beings, with schools and centers all over world.

Shayn Almeida is a DJ, yoga Instructor, audio engineer, and health and superfood specialist. He teaches Vinyasa Flow Yoga—Mixing Mind Body Spirit with Peace Love and BASS.

Shelly Prosko, PT, PYT, CPI, is a physical therapist and professional yoga therapist dedicated to empowering and educating individuals to create and sustain optimal health by teaching, promoting, and advocating for the integration of modern healthcare and yoga. She is a highly sought-after and respected pioneer of PhysioYoga, a combination of physical therapy and yoga therapy. Shelly guest-lectures at medical colleges; speaks internationally at conferences and events; offers on-site and online continuing education courses for healthcare professionals, yoga therapists, and yoga teachers; and offers workshops and individual PhysioYoga sessions for those suffering.

Sianna Sherman is an internationally renowned yoga teacher, community activator, and evocative storyteller, as well as a passionate speaker at festivals throughout the world. She is the founder of Rasa Yoga, Mythic Yoga Flow®, creator of the Goddess Yoga Project in partnership with *Yoga Journal*, and cofounder of Urban Priestess—a platform that serves the empowerment of women. Sianna was featured in *Yoga Journal* as one of the main teachers shaping the future of yoga. As a globe-trotting yogini, she offers high vibration gatherings, teacher trainings, workshops, sacred site retreats, and pilgrimages as an offering of Love. Sianna is an innovative, visionary spirit, with a deep devotion to Soul Alchemy. Her vision is to serve for the Benefit of All Beings and awaken magic into the world!

Stephanie Troy, LICSW, RYT, is a licensed clinical social worker, yoga teacher, nutrition coach, Reiki II practitioner, innovator, writer, and lover of enhancing authentic happiness. She is the owner of Your Whole Healing, which provides wellness counseling, yoga classes, nutrition education, and workshops. Her yoga project, Soba Yoga, was born from her career spanning over fifteen years in the area of addictions, corrections, and trauma. Practicing yoga since 2000, she has witnessed the calming affect it has had on her anxious mind. Stephanie has completed a 500-hour yoga teacher training with South Boston Yoga, Trauma Sensitive Yoga training through the Trauma Center at JRI, and Yin Yoga training with Josh Summers. Her blog, You and Me with Tea, is a composition of musings on health, wellness, yoga, and, well . . . tea. She is passionate about living, learning, and loving.

Sue Elkind is recognized internationally as a teacher's teacher, with over twenty-five years of yoga and studio ownership experience. Her in-depth knowledge of alignment and therapeutics, along with her passion to teach from her heart, allows her students to expand their potential both physically and spiritually. Sue is the director of DIG Yoga's 200- and 500-hour teacher training programs and is the author of *DIG Pregnancy, Birth & Baby: A Conscious and Empowered Approach to Prenatal and Postnatal Yoga*. She has also developed a Yoga Alliance 85-hour Pre/Post Natal Training that she teaches worldwide. Inspired by keeping great company, quality time in nature, and her loving family, Sue co-founded DIG Yoga with her husband, Naime Jezzeny, in Lambertville, New Jersey.

Tah Groen started teaching in 1997, when the yoga industry was just getting started. She loved yoga so much that it has been a significant part of her life since she was a teenager. Being an entrepreneur in business has always fascinated Tah, inspiring her to create an online membership program called Breath to Success, as well as to develop the Healing Touch Vinyasa Yoga Teacher Training program. Both are for yoga practitioners and yoga teachers looking to deepen their connection to self. Tah lives in San Diego with her partner of seventeen years and, besides her two adult daughters, has a rambunctious seven-year-old son.

Tanya Markul, is the cofounder/editor-in-chief at RebelleSociety.com and co-creator of RebelleWellness.com. She holds a BS in journalism and an MBA. In 2009, she became a certified yoga teacher. She has been practicing and studying with master teachers from all over the world, exploring and becoming deeply inspired by different traditions of yoga. She believes there is no greater class-room than life in this body, and the freedom of the present moment. She also believes life is a practice of discovery of individual nourishment, healing, and self-acceptance and is the most authentic creative expression of the self.

CONTRIBUTORS

Tara Judelle has experimented, for more than twenty-seven years, with all forms of movement flow, from dance to Tai Chi, to movement improvisation, and ultimately yoga. An English degree from Barnard College, post-graduate studies in theater directing, and a foray into screenwriting and directing brought her finally to the study of yoga and meditation. Certified originally in the Anusara method, Tara has taught yoga extensively, both nationally and internationally, for over twelve years. She has been a featured teacher as part of the Yogaglo team, allowing the yoga conversation to stream around the globe. In 2010, Tara moved from her home base in Los Angeles to direct a yoga program and retreat center in Bali, Indonesia, leading to her current schedule teaching workshops, retreats, and teacher trainings worldwide. Tara's classes focus on the discovery of embodied anatomy, bringing to the yogic tradition a scientific yet playful study of the movement vocabulary of the body and the ever-expanding perceptual awareness of the human mind.

Tymi Howard, E-RYT500, is an International Yoga Teacher, Certified Holistic Health Coach, owner of Guruv Yoga Studios in Orlando, Florida, and contributing writer for *Elephant Journal*. A teacher of teachers, she has been leading workshops and trainings for more than twenty-five years. Known for her artistic and dynamic teaching styles, Tymi is dedicated to inspiring people to discover and live out their life's purpose through the art of yoga. Join her in the yoga adventures on and off the mat in person, or online at YogaVibes.

Ulrica Norberg is a Swedish-born master yoga teacher with over twenty years of dedicated practice in yoga, meditation, and body therapy and holds a Master's degree in film and journalism. Ulrica has written over ten books, some of which have been translated into several languages. She leads trainings, workshops, and retreats around the world on a regular basis and is well known for her warmth, presence, and deep knowledge.

Valerie Goodman lives in Nashville, Tennessee. She teaches group classes and private clients with specific needs. She has acquired certification in Thai Yoga, Yoga for MS, and Yin Yoga. Continuous pursuit of knowledge is integrated in what and how she guides her students. Each class is taught with the intention to inspire self-awareness, build inner strength beyond the physical, and share the love. Valerie writes a blog about yoga and life and is working on writing her first book. In her spare time, she manages a dental office and helps nervous patients calm down with a few breaths and gentle moves.

Yulady Saluti never stops moving. She is a Yoga Alliance-certified yoga instructor who has appeared in DVDs and has rocked her yoga on television. She teaches at four different yoga studios and is doing all this while taking care of six kids and a devoted husband. After battling and overcoming a serious colorectal medical condition, Yulady dived headfirst into a new, healthy life, filled with yoga and studies in Ayurveda. It was only three years into her practice (and during her 20th surgery related to her former illness) that her doctors discovered she had Stage 2 breast cancer at the age of thirty-two. Yulady documented her journey as a mommy-yogi-with-cancer on her Youtube channel.